£12.50

C000131989

Obstetrics and Gynaecology

SERIES EDITORS

Ida Bromley MBE FCSP

Ida Bromely is a freelance consultant in London. From 1979–1986 she was the manager of the physiotherapy service for the Hampstead Health Authority in London. She has also worked in Australia, and for many years was in charge of physiotherapy at the Stoke Mandeville Hospital in England. She has lectured and run workshops in many countries including Turkey, U.S.A., South Africa and Australia, and written articles for several journals on subjects ranging from 'Rehabilitation of the Severely Disabled' to 'Problem Oriented Medical Recording and Audit'. She is also author of a well-known textbook, *Tetraplegia and Paraplegia*. From 1978–1982, she was Chairman of the Council of the Chartered Society of Physiotherapy. She is a past President of the Organisation of District Physiotherapists and currently President of the Society for Research in Rehabilitation.

Nancy Theilgaard Watts RPT PhD

Nancy Watts is Professor in the Physical Therapy Graduate Program of the MGH Institute of Health Professions at Massachusetts General Hospital in Boston. A physical therapy teacher for over 30 years, since 1965 most of her work has been in establishing advanced study programs for experienced therapists. Her major academic interests and publications concern methods of clinical teaching, economics of health care, and analysis of the process of judgment used by clinicians. Her clinical research has varied widely, ranging from studies of the effects of cold on spasticity to cost-effectiveness comparisons of different methods of treatment for common orthopaedic disorders. Dr Watts has served on a number of national and international commissions, and frequently teaches and consults in Britain, Scandinavia, and Latin America. She has also helped to prepare physical therapy teachers for schools in over 20 different countries.

VOLUME EDITOR

Julie McKenna MCSP

Julie McKenna is a leading member of the Association of Chartered Physiotherapists in Obstetrics and Gynaecology in England, and was chairman of this group from 1979–1982. She has worked as an obstetric physiotherapist since 1960, firstly in the Charing Cross Hospital Group and then at the Royal Free Hospital, both in London. She is particularly concerned with post-basic education. In 1981 she organised and taught on the first course in the speciality in Portugal. In 1983 she presented a paper at the Second European Congress of Obstetric Anaesthesia and Analgesia in Rome. She is the author of the chapter on Obstetrics in Cash's standard textbook for physiotherapists, part author of *You – After Childbirth* and contributes articles to various medical periodicals. She is at present a freelance lecturer and tutor and a member of the Education Subcommittee of the Association of Chartered Physiotherapists in Obstetrics and Gynaecology. She is married and has two sons.

INTERNATIONAL PERSPECTIVES IN PHYSICAL THERAPY 3

Obstetrics and Gynaecology

EDITED BY

Julie McKenna MCSP

Lecturer and Consultant.
Former Senior Obstetric Physiotherapist,
The Royal Free Hospital, London

CHURCHILL LIVINGSTONE
EDINBURGH LONDON MELBOURNE AND NEW YORK 1988

CHURCHILL LIVINGSTONE
Medical Division of Longman Group UK Limited

Distributed in the United States of America by
Churchill Livingstone Inc., 1560 Broadway, New
York, N.Y. 10036, and by associated companies,
branches and representatives throughout the world.

First published 1988

ISBN 0-443-03610-1

ISSN 0267-0380

British Library Cataloguing in Publication Data
Obstetrics and gynaecology. — (International
 perspective in physical therapy, ISSN 0267-0380; 3)
 1. Gynaecology 2. Obstetrics
 I. McKenna, Julie II. Series
 618   RG101

Library of Congress Cataloging in Publication Data
Obstetrics and gynaecology.
 (International perspectives in physical therapy; 3)
 Bibliography: p.
 Includes index.
 1. Gynecology. 2. Obstetrics. 3. Physical therapy.
I. McKenna, Julie. II. Series. [DNLM: 1. Genital
Diseases, Female. 2. Obstetrics. W1 IN827JM v.3/WQ
100 01453]
RG526.029   1988   618   87-25682

Produced by Longman Singapore Publishers (Pte) Ltd.
Printed in Singapore.

About the Series

The purpose of this series of books is to provide an international exchange of ideas and to explore different approaches in professional therapy practice.

The books will be written primarily for experienced clinicians. They are not intended as basic texts nor as reports on the most recent research, though elements of these aspects may be included.

Articles written by experts from a number of different countries will form the core of each volume. These will be supported by a commentary on the current 'state of the art' in the particular area of practice and an annotated bibliography of key references.

Each volume will cover a topic which we believe to be of universal interest. Some will be concerned with a troublesome symptom; others will be related to problems within a broad diagnostic category, for example sports injuries. Aspects of the organisation of practice and issues of professional concern will be the subjects of future books in the series.

In this volume we have adopted the convention of using 'she' for physiotherapist.

We hope that readers will let us have their reactions to the content and format of these publications. Suggestions of other topics considered to be of international interest which might provide the foci of future volumes would also be welcomed.

I.B.
N.T.W.

Preface

Although the title of this volume is 'Obstetrics and Gynaecology' it will be seen that obstetrics dominates. This is largely because it offers more scope to the physiotherapist. The important link between the two subjects is, however, emphasised in many of the chapters. The statement by Llewellyn Jones, 'Most teachers today agree that obstetrics and gynaecology form two intertwined branches of a single discipline', can be applied to physiotherapy as well as to medical practice. The specialist physiotherapist should be encouraged to view the cycle of a woman's life as a whole; good obstetric physiotherapy may, in many cases, affect later gynaecological outcome.

The speciality of physiotherapy in obstetrics and gynaecology is well established in the United Kingdom, but in many countries it is non-existent or comparatively new. This accounts for the disappointing response to world-wide enquiries for contributions to this volume. It is hoped that this addition to the series International Perspectives in Physical Therapy may help to remedy this situation and provide a stimulus to those already practising in the field.

London, 1988   J. McK.

Contributors

Glenys Culverwell MCSP
Teacher and Consultant in Relaxation Therapy. Former Senior Obstetric Physiotherapist, Bedford General Hospital, U.K.

Sheila M. Harrison MCSP MAPA
Assistant Principal Physiotherapist — Women's Health Department of Western Australia

Janette Krzyszton BAppSci (Phty) MAPA
Private Practice, Sydney, Australia

Helen Lawrence DipPhys FACP(O & G)
Private Practice, specialising in Obstetrics and Gynaecology, Hobart, Tasmania

Jill Mantle GradDipPhys MCSP DipTP
Senior Lecturer, The London Hospital School of Physiotherapy, The North East London Polytechnic, U.K.

Julie McKenna MCSP
Lecturer and Consultant. Former Senior Obstetric Physiotherapist, The Royal Free Hospital, London. Chairman of the Association of Chartered Physiotherapists in Obstetrics & Gynaecology 1979–1982, U.K.

Elizabeth Noble RPT
Director, Maternal & Child Health Center, Cambridge, MA, U.S.A. Former Chairwoman of the Obstetrics and Gynaecology section of the American Physical Therapy Association

Angela M. Shepherd MRCOG MD MCSP
Associate Specialist in Uro-gynaecology, Ham Green Hospital, Bristol, U.K.

Irene F. Skelton SRN SCM
Senior Midwife, The Queen Mother's Hospital, Glasgow. Midwifery Adviser to The International Society of Biophysical Medicine. Former Research Nurse, Southern General Hospital, Glasgow, U.K.

Myriam C.H. Vleminckx
Degrees in Physiotherapy and Physical Education from Leuven University, Belgium. Private Practice, specialising in Obstetrics and Aquatics, Belgium

Contents

Section One

1. Introduction   3
   Julie McKenna

2. Initiating a co-ordinated service in Western Australia   19
   Sheila Harrison

3. Sources of pain in labour   39
   Helen Lawrence

4. Maternal effort during labour and delivery   57
   Elizabeth Noble

5. Backache in pregnancy   69
   Jill Mantle

6. Aspects of body learning for the childbearing year   93
   Glenys Culverwell and Julie McKenna

7. Pregnancy and recovery: the aquatic approach   107
   Myriam Vleminckx

8. Two non-pharmacological forms of pain relief in labour
   Part 1. Acupuncture   129
   Irene Skelton
   Part 2. Transcutaneous electrical nerve stimulation   141
   Janette Krzyszton

9. Urinary incontinence and the pelvic floor   151
   Angela Shepherd

Section Two

Annotated bibliography   177

Index   187

SECTION ONE

Introduction

HISTORY OF PHYSIOTHERAPY IN OBSTETRICS AND GYNAECOLOGY

It is probable that the oldest speciality in physical medicine is in the area of obstetrics; its origins date from the late 1920s in the United Kingdom. Since much of the practice in the subject overseas stems from the pioneer work in this country, it seems appropriate in an international volume to trace this early history. And since this situation prevails to this day — most recently (1981) an English physiotherapist was invited to organise the first course and initiate the speciality in Portugal — it would also seem useful to include details of the system of post-registration education in the United Kingdom.

Obstetric physiotherapy owes much to the fact that in the late 1920s the obstetrician in charge of the unit at St Thomas' Hospital was Dr Fairbairn who valued the postnatal physiotherapy already operating there and was the first to suggest extending the scope to include antenatal treatment. This suggestion accorded with the ideas of Minnie Randell (herself a midwife and a physiotherapist) who was superintendent of the Department and School of Physiotherapy at St Thomas' Hospital at that time. She had been giving postnatal exercises for many years and was beginning to realise that she could help her mothers to recover more quickly in the postnatal period if she saw them before the birth. Today's practitioners are well aware of this important link and that the foundations of postnatal rehabilitation are best laid antenatally. In Chapter 6 it is shown how prenatal education in body awareness has far reaching benefits in the puerperium and after. Together with the physician Dr Kathleen Vaughan, Minnie Randell started antenatal classes teaching exercises and relaxation as well as education in the events of childbirth. They were helped by Margaret Morris, a professional dancer who is alleged to have said on seeing her first delivery 'Why wasn't the mother rehearsed?'. All three of these women wrote books on aspects of the subject and Minnie Randell's *Training for Childbirth* in particular remained the textbook for those working in the speciality for many years. Anyone consulting it today might be surprised to find incorporated many of our 'new' ideas such as postures for the first stage of labour and stretching exercises to prepare for delivery. At the 1921 Congress of the Chartered Society of Massage and Medical Gymnastics, later to become the Chartered Society of Physiotherapy (CSP), Dr Fairbairn stated in his lecture: 'Nothing inhibits uterine action so much as emotional symptoms. There is no attitude of mind which enables a woman to deliver herself naturally so much as that of complete confidence in herself as a physically strong and healthy woman.'

In the 1930s the obstetrician Grantly Dick-Read considered the effect of the emotions on the pain felt by the labouring woman. He maintained that fear leads to tension which in turn leads to pain and increased fear. He sought to break this cycle by teaching relaxation (which was already included in Minnie Randell's programme) and by educating the expectant woman in the events of labour. Dick-Read's method and success (the latter no doubt due in some part to the fact that he himself prepared and delivered his clients) received wide publicity, although in medical circles he remained a somewhat controversial figure. This was partly due to a misrepresentation of his views; he never taught 'painless childbirth' but rather 'childbirth without fear', and revised editions of his book of that title have remained in print. The physiotherapist Helen Heardman based her teaching on Dick-Read's ideas and became one of a group to form the first Obstetric Association of Physiotherapists in 1948. Their aim was to exchange views and experiences, and very soon they instigated the first specialised courses at Leeds Maternity Hospital which included attendance at deliveries.

In the 1950s a new trend reached Britain from Russia via Paris — psychoprophylaxis. The term, meaning 'mind prevention', is based on the theory of Pavlov's conditioned reflex. Its followers suggested that women felt pain in labour because they were conditioned to do so by history — 'I will greatly multiply thy sorrow and thy conception' (Genesis II, 16) and more strongly in the New English Bible — 'I will increase your labour and your groaning'. The aim was to de-condition the woman and teach her to associate contractions in labour not with pain but with acquired skills, such as special breathing patterns and self-massage, and by a process of distraction to block the pain pathways to the brain.

It was a very rigid form of training incorporating controlled patterns of breathing, and although doubtless it helped some women, for many it tended to augment rather than allay anxiety. It was somewhat inflexible and therefore ill-adapted to the unpredictability of labour, and many midwives found it interfered with the desired communication between them and the labouring women. In 1963 a physiologist working in Bristol, R. St John Buxton, in a study of respiration in labour, compared the effects of different types of antenatal training. In the group trained in the psychoprophylaxis method he found that most stages of labour were characterised by hyperventilation. Studies in Oxford by John Stradling (1983) suggest the inadvisability of encouraging methods which cause over-breathing in labour, which may prove harmful to an already compromised fetus. *The New Childbirth* by Erna Wright published in 1964 expounding psychoprophylaxis achieved wide publicity, and this method is still practised in many places today. It is obviously important for physiotherapists to study the results of research by physiologists into respiration in labour.

In 1961 with a membership of over 100, the name of the Association was changed to The Obstetric Association of Chartered Physiotherapists, and during the following years a standard syllabus was drawn up for courses which were being run in several centres in the country. In 1978 gynaecology was added to the speciality and the name Association of Chartered Physiotherapists in Obstetrics and Gynaecology (ACPOG) was adopted. This addition was largely due to the work and enthusiasm of Dorothy Mandelstam (a physiotherapist with an international reputation as a continence adviser), Sheila Harrison (who has since emigrated to Australia and contributed a chapter to this volume) and the obstetrician/gynaecologist John Carron Brown (at that time president of the Association). In 1984 the ACPOG Course became a validated and certificated post-registration course of the CSP (Chartered Society of Physiotherapy).

THE ASSOCIATION OF CHARTERED PHYSIOTHERAPISTS IN OBSTETRICS AND GYNAECOLOGY

The Association is managed by an executive committee elected by the membership and headed by a chairman. The president is usually a distinguished obstetrician/gynaecologist; an Education Subcommittee is responsible for areas described on page 6. There are three categories of Membership of the Association. Full membership is open to annually subscribing members of the CSP who have successfully completed the post-registration requirements of the Association; provisional membership is available to those working towards full membership; and honorary membership is offered to members of professional bodies at the discretion of the executive committee. Other members of the medical, paramedical and nursing professions may become Associates of the Association. A study weekend is held annually, the Association's Journal is issued twice yearly and literature is available from the Book Secretary. In some areas regular workshop groups are organised by local members.

POST-REGISTRATION EDUCATION FOR MEMBERSHIP OF ACPOG

As the course has been validated and certified by the CSP, those working for membership must be annually subscribing members of the Society. They must also have had a minimum of two years general experience since qualification. The course is in two parts: a foundation (Part I) which is for full membership of ACPOG and an advanced (Part II) for those wishing to study the subject more deeply.* Candidates for Part I attend a six day course at an approved centre and within two years present a written submission which includes evidence of having undertaken a prescribed practical module. In the obstetric section the submission should include the aims and objectives of antenatal physiotherapy, schemes of classes for antenatal and postnatal women, as well as an account of individual treatments. The candidate must show a sensitivity to the needs of parents-to-be and the very particular needs of special cases such as the unmarried and teenagers. In the gynaecological section she is expected to demonstrate an awareness of the emotional aspect of patients with gynaecological problems and the physiotherapist's role in the unit. In both sections an account is needed of the place of the physiotherapist in the team and how she works with the other members. Included with the dissertation must be evidence of having fulfilled all the practical requirements (the Association issues special forms to facilitate this). Throughout the preparation of the presentation the candidate is advised to be in continual

---

* Since October 1987 the designations Part I and Part II have been dropped. (Ed.)

communication with her tutor who will guide and monitor progress. The written submission is examined by two assessors who are members of the Education Subcommittee. If both agree that a satisfactory standard has been achieved, the candidate is accepted for membership. If there is disagreement or if both agree on a failure, the submission goes to the chairman of the Education Subcommittee who may recommend further work to be done.

The Part II course is designed to enable members to broaden and deepen their knowledge, possibly with a view to taking part in research and helping in the running of the Association. The first such course was held at the London Hospital in 1984, and it is proposed that one shall be organised each year. The course consists of six study days followed by an examination paper (set and marked by the relevant specialist course lecturers) to be completed by the candidate within the six weeks following.

THE SPECIALITY TODAY IN THE UNITED KINGDOM

In January 1987 there were 297 full members of ACPOG (of which 31 were resident overseas) and 228 provisional members and associates. The physiotherapist works as part of the obstetric and gynaecological team attending ward rounds, clinics and medical consultative meetings. If there is an Incontinence Clinic in the unit she may be involved with the medical and nursing staff in urodynamic investigations. In a teaching hospital she may lecture to medical students, midwives, nurses and physiotherapists. She may have less experienced physiotherapists working for her who need clinical teaching. If her department is considered a suitable centre for training prospective ACPOG members she may act as tutor or clinical superviser, guiding the candidate through the practical work needed for her submission. In some larger centres (six at present in the United Kingdom) there may be an annual ACPOG training course which she will organise with the help of other members of the Association.

In the obstetric department the physiotherapist will work as a member of the team in the preparation for parenthood, organising on her own or with the midwife the programme of classes, and co-ordinating input with other members of the team. The specific role of the physiotherapist will be to care for the physical problems of the pregnant woman as they arise, but where possible to obviate them by teaching preventive measures. Her role also includes participating in a training for labour programme in co-operation with the midwife, and being present in the labour ward if called upon to support her mothers. It is important for her to see the outcome of the training programmes and be continually in touch with labour ward procedures. Frequently the course may include a postnatal reunion class giving the physiotherapist the opportunity to assess recovery and give further help where needed. In the hospital she will look after the postnatal ward giving treatments individually and in groups.

Childbirth is one of the most important events in a woman's life. With higher living standards (at least for some members of the community) and with improved antenatal care and technology (such as antenatal screening), childbirth has become a relatively safe event for mother and baby. The concern for safety has been replaced by a concern for the quality of the experience on the part of the woman. While wishing primarily for a healthy baby, she also wants to be involved, as far as safety permits, in her own labour and delivery and to be fulfilled by it. Apart from the important physical aspects of preparation, the emotional preparation can have a great influence on her feelings about the event. The physiotherapist must be ready to encourage positive thinking but at the same time in some cases to damp down a too high expectation of her achievement which may lead to a sense of failure as described in Chapter 4 by Noble. This requires a great sensitivity on the part of the physiotherapist and an empathy with the members of her antenatal class. Good communication skills are essential for those specialising in this care.

In gynaecology, daily duties will include responsibility for the physiotherapy requirements on the gynaecological wards, paying particular attention to the special needs of these patients, which differ from those of patients undergoing general surgery in two main ways. Firstly, owing to the high vascularity of the pelvic region they are particularly susceptible to circulatory problems. Secondly, the very nature of their condition and the surgery required causes strong emotional and psychological reactions of which the specialist physiotherapist will be aware. Outpatient referrals from the gynaecologist and the general practioner will also be treated. Treatments may include pulsed shortwave for pelvic inflammatory disease and exercise and/or electrical treatment for stress incontinence. The latter may form the greatest proportion of her work and be the most rewarding (Ch. 9).

THE PROBLEMS OF THE SPECIALITY IN THE UNITED KINGDOM TODAY

The main problem is that there are not enough ACPOG members to supply the ever-growing demand for antenatal and postnatal classes: as it is, many members work only part-time. The situation was highlighted recently in the results of a project presented by an undergraduate student in physiotherapy at the London Hospital. A questionaire was sent to every Health District in the British Isles asking for information regarding types of classes and personnel involved. The data applied to a specific week in 1984 when the number of members of ACPOG was 280. 85.7% replied giving particulars of 2283 classes in the community and hospitals. The physiotherapy input was 79% in the hospital situation and 37% in the community. On these statistics it seems unlikely that there will ever be enough members to supply the demand, at least in the community. In addition, in scattered communities in rural areas it might seem an uneconomical use of the physiotherapist's time. The survey revealed that the person most commonly involved in taking classes was the midwife, and that in the majority of community classes she worked without a physiotherapist. This has long been known and has given rise to the need for the midwife to be taught some basic skills by the physiotherapist. For many years senior members of the Association have taken part in the instruction in Teaching for Preparation for Parenthood courses organised by the Royal College of Midwives. However, it is appreciated by all that this arrangement cannot hope to enable a midwife to provide the same level of care in this respect as the obstetric physiotherapist. Discussion is currently taking place within the Association relating to the objectives of such teaching and the standards to be aimed at; a syllabus is being prepared for use throughout the United Kingdom. During 1986/7 members of the Royal College of Midwives, the Health Visitors Association and ACPOG have had regular meetings to discuss and define their different roles in the education for parenthood. They have drawn up a statement of good practice which has been endorsed by the CSP. Since it gives an indication of how the three professions work together — each employing their special skills but all in harmony with one another — it is included here.

STATEMENT BY THE ROYAL COLLEGE OF MIDWIVES, THE HEALTH VISITORS' ASSOCIATION AND THE CHARTERED SOCIETY OF PHYSIOTHERAPY ON WORKING TOGETHER IN PSYCHOPHYSICAL PREPARATION FOR CHILDBIRTH

1. Midwives, health visitors and obstetric physiotherapists take part in providing education in preparation for childbirth and parenthood. This is an important form of preventive medicine and health education and parents derive maximum benefit where a team approach operates.

2. The role of the midwife is that of the practitioner of normal midwifery, caring for the women within the hospital and community throughout the continuum of pregnancy, childbirth and the puerperium. She has an important contribution to make in health education, counselling and support. In this context her aim is to facilitate the realisation of the woman's potential in mothering by encouraging her to express needs, discuss expectations and air anxieties. She has the responsibility of monitoring the woman's physical, psychological and social wellbeing and is in a unique position to be able to correlate parent education with midwifery care.

3. The role of the health visitor in this field is to offer advice to the parents-to-be on the many health and social implications of birth and the development of the child. She is in a very special position in the family scene to inform them of the services available and to encourage them to use them. She can also reinforce the advice given by the obstetric physiotherapist and midwife.

4. The role of the obstetric physiotherapist is to help a woman adjust to the physical changes throughout pregnancy and the puerperium so that stress may be minimised. She will assess and treat any skeletal and muscular problems such as backache. She is a skilled teacher of effective relaxation, breathing awareness and positioning and thus helps to prepare the woman for labour. In the postnatal period she will give advice on physical activity, teach postnatal exercises and where necessary give specialised treatments.

5. In order for the services of the team to be of maximum benefit to parents there should be a close liaison among its members. Shared learning sessions should take place to help to ensure that techniques and advice are consistent, related to current practice and meet the needs of parents. The midwife, health visitor and obstetric physiotherapist should be in regular contact and should operate an effective referral system.

January 1987

CHALLENGES

1. Prophylaxis

The involvement of the physiotherapist specialising in obstetrics and gynaecology in a woman's life usually starts in the antenatal period, when the expectant mother books in for preparation classes. In these she will be taught about her body and the changes taking place in it, be helped to minimise the stresses of pregnancy and learn the best ways of managing her labour. It is becoming increasingly obvious that this is too late — that she can be helped much more if she has the advice of the physiotherapist at a much earlier stage in her life. It is the preventive aspect of the speciality that enforces this view — a view expressed in several of the chapters in this book. Mantle (Ch. 5) suggests that backcare should be promoted in Well Women's Clinics or even earlier, in the schools. Shepherd (Ch. 9) describes incontinence as being largely a condition of the Western world. She cites the difference between English women of whom only 40% in a trial using a perionometer were able to produce a measureable pressure by a pelvic floor contraction, and a group of Malay and Chinese with a score of 95%. This is attributed in part to the fact that mothers of girls in the latter races teach their daughters at puberty to perform pelvic floor exercises and so prepare them to become satisfactory marital partners. We should learn from this and again see our role broadened to encompass pre-conceptual training or, better still, training in girls' schools. Another possibility is to enthuse our expectant mothers so that they teach their daughters. As things are at present, women are seen for the first time when both backs and pelvic floor are potentially disadvantaged by the pregnancy. Culverwell and McKenna (Ch. 6) emphasise the improved general lifestyle resulting from an exercise programme which is not directed exclusively towards pregnancy. With the interest today in good health, exercise and pre-conceptual care there are opportunities for the specialist physiotherapist to help women long before they appear in the antenatal clinic. This help should affect not only the childbearing period but also the long term gynaecological outlook for the woman.

2. Education

The speciality of physiotherapy in obstetrics and gynaecology is unusual in that there has never been more than a minimal coverage of the subjects in the basic physiotherapy training. Education has therefore been a prime concern from the 1930s, when the small pioneer group met to discuss their new interest, to the present day with its structured courses. These courses are planned and monitored by the Education Subcommittee who submit all details of programmes and lecturers to the CSP. A network of trained tutors and clinical supervisers guide candidates through their practical work and written submission.

The shortage of ACPOG members and the consequent need for a syllabus for training midwives in some of the physical skills have already been mentioned. Sundry other matters are dealt with by the Education Subcommittee, such as designing patient hand-outs for use by the membership, arranging book lists and monitoring relevant articles of interest from medical journals. The Subcommittee is aware of the need for continual up-dating of the educational aspects of the Association, realising that good education leads to improved patient care. They are also sensitive to the importance of fostering working relationships with other members of the health care team by sharing in educational projects and by encouraging them to become Associates of ACPOG.

3. Research

Elements of the speciality are ever-changing, especially the obstetric component, and the physiotherapist should be aware of current research, as well as initiating or contributing to investigations herself. Many changes in the practice of physiotherapy have taken place as a result of research. It has already been noted how the studies of St John Buxton and later Stradling led to modifications in the teaching of breathing for labour. The work of Flynn et al (1978) and Russell (1982) has led to the interest in mobility in labour and upright delivery positions which has resulted in the need for training in different postures and stretching exercises antenatally as described in Chapter 6. Further research projects are needed, such as that described by Lawrence, to assess the results of various training programmes. In the gynaecological unit, treatment of stress incontinence is given by exercise and/or interferential currents (said to stimulate the involuntary component of the pelvic floor). However, the evidence of the efficacy of the latter is so far not convincing and further studies are needed.

A potential strength of the specialist physiotherapist is that she sees women both in the obstetric and gynaecological units and is thus in a position to study the long-term effects of the management of the childbearing period. This presents invaluable opportunities for research and evaluation. A random sample of 86 cases of pelvic floor laxity referred to the physiotherapist for treatment at the Royal Free Hospital, London in 1986/87, revealed that all but 7 were parous women. This is an example of an opening for interesting investigation on the following lines: what was the significant factor — was it the pregnancy itself, the management of or type of delivery, the fact of having or not having had ante and/or postnatal exercise? How was it related to the practice of episiotomy? There are obstetricians who think that prolonged pushing in the second stage is damaging to the supportive ligaments of the uterus and that an episiotomy can prevent this and give a better final result. It will be interesting to see whether the upright delivery positions will result in long-term benefit to the pelvic floor muscles. All these points should concern the physiotherapist and may have a direct bearing on her work. The following chain of events underlines the significance of obstetric procedures to the physiotherapist working in the gynaecological unit: the use of epidural anaesthesia in labour increases the forceps rate (Bates and Helm 1985) — a forceps delivery increases the risk of damage to the pelvic floor (Snooks et al 1984) and the consequent need for physiotherapy (either in the long or short term) for the pelvic muscle laxity.

4. Promotion

Wherever possible physiotherapists should attend national and international meetings relevant to the speciality. An excellent platform in recent years has been the European Congress of Obstetric Anaesthesia and Analgesia. This is a multi-disciplinary forum and ACPOG members have contributed papers at the three meetings which have so far been held. There are still areas of ignorance, especially in the medical profession, as to the speciality and members should wherever possible take part in teaching programmes for medical students. A recent letter from an ACPOG member in a medical journal on the treatment of stress incontinence brought dozens of letters of enquiry from general practitioners throughout the country. However, ultimately it is the standard of work of the individual which is the best promotion of the speciality.

CONTRIBUTIONS TO THIS VOLUME

A major challenge to members of the obstetric team is the relief of pain in labour. Childbirth in the United Kingdom today may be safer than it has ever been, but there is still a search for the perfect form of pain relief which gives satisfaction to the woman without compromising the neonate. Programmes of antenatal training (psychophysical) aim to increase the pain tolerance by educating women in the events of labour and teaching relaxation. In her chapter, Lawrence analyses the causes of pain in labour and describes a research project she undertook in Hobart, Tasmania. A sample of 338 primiparous women took part in the study, two-thirds of whom had had prenatal training. Pain measurement was done using an adaptation of the McGill Pain Questionaire and the Visual Analogue Scale. As has been found in previous studies (Davenport-Slack and Boylan 1974, Sternbach 1968) the prepared women showed no decrease in the incidence of pain but a better control by the women resulted and a reduction in the need for analgesia.

The last ten or so years have seen many changes in the management of labour based in part on the work of researchers and in part on the demands of parents-to-be. Noble outlines these changes and how they should affect the attitudes of childbirth educators. To some it may seem that she is preaching to the converted — certainly many units in the United Kingdom are already practising the methods she publicises. But there still remain areas in this and other countries where imposed breathing patterns are encouraged and the labouring woman is still to be found flat on her back in the delivery room.

Culverwell and McKenna outline a training programme to achieve body awareness and fitness for pregnancy, birth and the postnatal period. This includes posture, exercise and relaxation which can benefit all women besides being specifically directed towards pain tolerance in labour. The Active Birth Movement is discussed and the special training required for it. The importance of this care being undertaken by professionals is underlined in view of the vulnerability of the woman's body during the childbearing period.

Antenatal instruction should include an account of the various forms of pain relief available and their effects. While realising that she may need some help with the pain in addition to her relaxation training, today's expectant mother is anxious about how this may affect herself and the baby. It is known that pethidine affects the baby adversely (Redshaw and Rosenblatt 1982), and that epidural anaesthesia, by causing a decrease in the oxytocin output in the second stage of labour, increases the forceps rate (Bates and Helm 1985). Some form of pain relief is needed which allows the woman to remain in control, able to co-operate in her delivery and remain mobile for as long as possible. TENS and acupuncture may answer these needs and are becoming increasingly popular.

The CSP has approved the practice of acupuncture which is now part of the physiotherapist's repertoire in the United Kingdom, and regular postgraduate courses are held in the subject. It seems particularly appropriate that the obstetric physiotherapist should be involved in its use in labour. Meanwhile this contribution by a midwife is especially welcome. Skelton has had wide experience in its use, has contributed articles on the subject to various journals including the *Midwives Chronicle* and the *ACPOG Journal* and teaches it to midwives and physiotherapists. She gives the result of her pilot study undertaken at the Southern General Hospital, Glasgow.

TENS has been used by physiotherapists for many years for the relief of chronic pain. According to Krzyszton, in her history of its use in labour, it was first reported in Russia in 1971. It has the advantage of allowing the labouring woman to stay mobile (which if there are no medical contra-indications is encouraged in many units today), while having no known side-effects on her or her baby. The fact that the woman operates the machine herself, controlling the output, gives her added reassurance and satisfaction. The writer summarises some of the studies done on its use and describes the method of application. She rightly underlines the necessity for careful antenatal instruction to both parents. She also states the need for all members of the obstetric team to be conversant with every aspect of the machine and its usage.

It was hoped to include a section on hypnosis for labour in this chapter. Details of a study were received from Holland, but unfortunately it was too small to be regarded as a significant contribution to the subject. It was, however, interesting to learn that the method is being tried there and no doubt more data will become available in the future. In the United Kingdom a randomised trial undertaken at St George's Hospital Medical School, London (1986) on self-hypnosis in labour revealed a more satisfied mother than in the control group but no difference in the relief of pain. As in a similar study by Charles et al (1978), labour was longer in the hypnotised group. Further studies are needed and would be interesting in the light of the continual search for non-invasive pain relief.

When asked by prospective mothers about exercise in pregnancy, physiotherapists have long given the response 'swimming and walking', as these two non-competitive activities require no force or strain. Recently, obstetric physiotherapists have started special pool sessions as part of antenatal health training. Vleminckx describes the formation of the Association Nationale Natation et Maternité in France involving midwives, doctors, physiotherapists and swimming instructors in 1977, and how the Association has spread to many countries since that time. The positive as well as enjoyable effects of swimming are described with antenatal and postnatal programmes of activities in the water. These include possibilities for the non-swimmer as well as the experienced swimmer, and she illustrates her chapter with photographs showing the various exercises. This could be a useful blueprint for anyone setting up a similar service.

It has been said that an important aspect of obstetric physio-therapy is in the realm of preventive medicine. This is nowhere more apparent than in the consideration of backache in pregnancy. In her chapter, Mantle analyses the causes of backache in pregnancy and how it may be prevented, suggesting that prophylactic care should, if possible, start before conception. She proceeds to discuss the various remedies for backache in pregnancy, under-lining the necessity for careful assessment before treatment. Back-ache is the commonest problem of pregnancy and can colour adversely what should be an enjoyable period in a woman's life. For too long it has been accepted by many members of the medical profession as an inevitable symptom of pregnancy — the physio-therapist with her general training and the added post-registration training in obstetrics must rise to the challenge of this sometimes crippling condition.

Since the subject of gynaecology became part of the speciality in 1978 members of ACPOG have become increasingly involved in the treatment and management of incontinence. Dr Shepherd was a physiotherapist before she studied medicine and then specialised in urology. In her chapter she describes normal bladder function and how pregnancy and labour affect it. She enumerates the different types of incontinence, which is the main area for the physiotherapist. She describes preventive measures and gives an account of the re-education of the pelvic floor by physiotherapeutic means. It is hoped that physiotherapists will increasingly concern themselves both in the treatment of this distressing condition, and in research into its causes.

It would appear that the claim that physiotherapy in obstetrics and gynaecology as a speciality originated in the United Kingdom, is valid. That the speciality flourishes in many other countries today is frequently due to the pioneer work of visiting physiotherapists from the United Kingdom. However, there are places where it is still not developed, and physiotherapists continue to be invited from the United Kingdom to instigate it. In view of this it seemed particularly interesting to have a chapter on a new development in Western Australia. The scale of the area and problem was unusual, but the principles apply to any situation where a service is being set up. Harrison was an active member and former chairman of ACPOG before emigrating to Australia, so was well versed in the educational aspect of the speciality. In her chapter can be found a syllabus of post-registration education in obstetrics and gynaecology for physiotherapists similar to that in use in the United Kingdom, and an assessment of the needs and problems which faced her. She emphasises the importance of continual monitoring of courses — essential for the maintenance of standards. Finally and most importantly, she shows an awareness of the necessity of involving other members of the obstetric and gynaecological teams in the educational programme. This chapter offers useful guidelines which can be applied to similar situations whatever the scale of the undertaking.

This book is intended to encourage the specialist physiotherapist to re-assess her work and (where necessary) modify it in the light of current thought and research. It is by this means that she will prove herself an essential member of the obstetric and gynaecological team.

REFERENCES

Bates R G, Helm C W 1985 Epidural analgesia during labour. Why does this increase the forceps delivery rate? Journal of The Royal Society of Medicine 78: 890–892

Buxton St J 1965 Maternal respiration in labour. Obstetric Association of Physiotherapists' publication.

Charles A G, Norr K L, Block C R, Meyering G, Meyers E 1978 Obstetric and psychological effects of psychoprophylactic preparation for childbirth. American Journal of Gynaecology 131: 44–52

Davenport-Slack B, Boyland S H 1974 Psychological correlates of childbirth pain. Psychosomatic Medicine 36 (3): 215–223

Dick-Read G 1969 Childbirth without fear, 5th edn. Pan Books Ltd, London

Fairbairn J S 1922 Physical treatment in obstetrics and gynaecology. Journal of the Chartered Society of Massage and Medical Gymnastics 7 (10)

Flynn A M, Kelly J, Hollins G, Lynch P F 1978 Ambulation in labour. British Medical Journal 2: 591–593

Llewellyn-Jones D 1986 Fundamentals of obstetrics and gynaecology, 4th edn, vol II, p 15. Faber & Faber, London

Randell M 1945 Training for childbirth. J & A Churchill, London

Redshaw M, Rosenblatt D B 1982 The influence of analgesia in labour on the baby. Midwife Health Visitor & Community Nurse 18 (4): 126–132

Russell J G B 1982 The rationale of primitive delivery positions. British Journal of Obstetrics & Gynaecology 89: 7I2–7I5

Snooks S J, Swash M, Setchell M, Henry M M 1984 Injury to innervation of pelvic floor sphincter musculature in childbirth. Lancet 2: 546–550

St George's Hospital Medical School 1986 Randomised trial of self-hypnosis for analgesia in labour. British Medical Journal 292: 657–658

Stradling J 1983 Respiratory physiology in labour. Journal of The Association of Chartered Physiotherapists in Obstetrics & Gynaecology 53: 5–7

Sternbach R A 1968 Pain: a psychophysiological analysis. Academic Press, New York.

Initiating a co-ordinated service in Western Australia

When considering any aspect of service provision in Western Australia the immense size of the area is worthy of attention.

It is the largest state in Australia and makes up nearly one third of the continent. It has an area of 2 525 500 sq km, approximately 11 times the size of mainland United Kingdom. The population numbers 1 400 000, of whom 74% live in the capital Perth or the remainder of the South West region (Fig. 2.1).

The physiotherapy section of the Health Department of Western Australia is managed by a Principal and four Assistant Principal Physiotherapists. Each Assistant has special interest, experience and expertise in one aspect of physiotherapy and is responsible for the provision of a service in that speciality throughout the State.

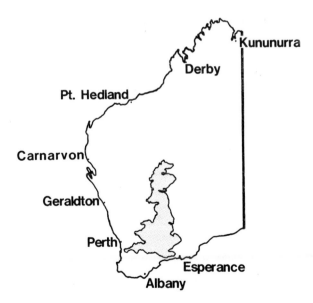

Fig. 2.1 Western Australia and the United Kingdom.

Table 2.1 Establishment of physiotherapists and numbers working in obstetrics and gynaecology in the State

Employer	Total	Staff Obstetrics & gynaecology
Health department		
Central administration	5	1
Metropolitan area		
— hospitals and health centres	32	32
— community staff	33	
— special schools	4	
Country areas		
— hospitals and health centres	71	71
Total	145	104
Other agencies		
WAIT*	20	3
Public teaching hospitals	207	9
(affiliated to Health Dept.)		
Total	227	12
Overall total	372	116

In addition to these figures there are a further 558 Registered Physiotherapists in the State of whom approximately 105 are in full time private practice.

*The Western Australian Institute of Technology, now designated Curtin University of Technology

Obstetrics and gynaecology is one of these and is alternatively entitled Women's Health. The position was created in October 1984 and to date is the only such appointment in Australia.

The Health Department has an establishment of 144 physiotherapists. The disposition of all the physiotherapists in the State and their input to obstetrics and gynaecology is shown in Table 2.1

THE ASSIGNMENT

The assignment was to introduce a progressive co-ordinated programme of physiotherapy in obstetrics and gynaecology which would be of a uniformly high standard and capitalise on the expertise already available.

Implementation

1. To conduct training workshops
2. To compile a procedure manual for staff guidance
3. To visit throughout the State to monitor the implementation of the programme and give assistance where necessary.

Aims of the procedure manual

1. To give a basic core of practical and theoretical knowledge to enable the therapist to commence work in an accurate and effective manner.
2. To provide a range of reference material, to encourage the growth of confidence and expertise.
3. To form the resource base for a co-ordinated programme in obstetrics and gynaecology throughout the State.

THE SERVICE IN THE PAST

This varied throughout the State according to the staff members' interest in the subject, past experience, existing service and encouragement from local doctors and midwives.

At a student level obstetrics and gynaecology is a small or even optional part of the syllabus, with little practical experience to be gained. Thus most knowledge and expertise has to be acquired after registration, in the form of post-registration courses or post-graduate diplomas.

THE CHALLENGE

Physiotherapy in obstetrics and gynaecology is a professional health care discipline devoted to the care of women. It has progressed from primary therapy during the lying-in period to a comprehensive programme of preventative, curative and palliative medicine from the menarche to old age.

The development of this discipline is centred on meeting the needs of the childbearing population in Western Australia. During the period 1972 to 1983 some well-established trends have emerged as confirmed in Table 2.2.

The key factor in these figures is the fertility rate. This index was in excess of 100 prior to 1972; since then it has slowly declined to the levels quoted; it appears to have stabilised.

Whilst the number of females aged 15–44 has continued to increase at a rate greater than that of the total population, the number of births has risen but at a reduced rate.

On this evidence it is realistic to predict the birth rate will continue to rise. This will be subject to a stable fertility rate and the continued growth in the number of females in the 15–44 age group.

Table 2.2 Demographic table — birth and fertility rates. (Source: Maternal & Child Health in W.A 1968–1983 Health Dept.)

Item	1977	1982	1977/1982 % change	1983	1982/1983 % change
Total population	1 197 089	1 336 911	+ 11.7	1 364 455	+ 2.1
Females Age15–44	267–231	313 275	+ 17.2	321 121	+ 2.5
Total births	20 835	22 339	+ 7.2	23 013	+ 3.0
Fertility rate (births/1000 females)	78.0	71.3		71.6	

CLINICAL PROGRAMMES

Most of the ante and postnatal programmes take the form of group therapy, but are easily adapted for use with a couple or one person. Individual assessment and treatments are an essential part of physiotherapy in obstetrics and gynaecology. An outline of the clinical programmes is as follows:

Women in hospital

Obstetrics

Antenatal — Long stay patients will have individual programmes to retain their fitness and prepare for labour.

Postnatal — Post-operative care after anaesthesia. Exercise and advice programmes to promote restoration to full function and facilitate the change to their new role. Individual therapy to local trauma.

Gynaecology

— Pre- and post-operative care to reduce the effects of anaesthesia, promote recovery by general and specific exercises.

— Advice on activity and rest at home and the gradual return to full function.

Women at home

Obstetrics — preparation for childbirth groups

There are advantages in having separate groups for primigravid and multigravid women as their needs vary widely.

Primigravid groups are divided into three categories:

1. For couples
2. For unaccompanied women
3. For teenagers.

Multigravid groups

Consist of singles and couples together. Antenatal courses vary in length from 6–8 sessions to intensive short courses of 3–4 sessions for late bookers into classes or multigravid women. Ideally, pregnant couples need to prepare for their role together and both attend every class. This normally creates a need for couples' classes to be held in the evening, but timing is matched to community needs as shift work is common in mining towns.

Owing to the increasing demand for classes, physiotherapists are often under pressure to accept large numbers of couples in antenatal groups. Classes should be limited to 10 or 12 couples to facilitate the learning of physical skills, enhance group dynamics and improve client satisfaction. The drop-out rate is high in classes that are too large.

General practitioners and hospital staff are given information stressing that early booking is the only way to obtain the present service. Administrators are advised that expansion will be required to satisfy the demand effectively.

Obstetric fitness groups

1. Physiotherapy healthy pregnancy class — for women from 12 weeks to term.
2. Physiotherapy postnatal class — for women and their babies from six weeks to six months postpartum.

MONITORING THE SERVICE

The extent of the implementation of the clinical programmes described in this text varies throughout the State. As the physiotherapists' awareness of women's needs grows and their own knowledge and expertise increases, the scope of the work is gradually being expanded. This is subject to the usual constraints of pressure on staff time. Contact with staff is maintained by:

— Monthly reports
— Telephone
— Visits by assistant principal physiotherapists
— Senior staff meetings in Perth
— Annual Conference of Health Department staff.

Visits

Outside the metropolitan area of Perth visits are generally planned to include several physiotherapy departments over a period of two or more days. The great distances to be covered make it possible to use a car only for visits within three or four hours' drive of Perth.

Travel to other parts of the State is therefore by air and covers many hundreds of kilometres; the size of the planes can vary considerably too (Fig. 2.2).

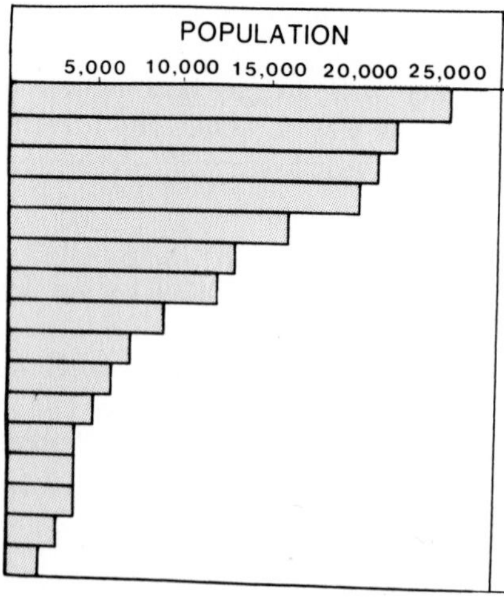

POPULATION 5,000 10,000 15,000 20,000 25,000	TOWN	Kms FROM PERTH	STAFF
	ROCKINGHAM	45	3
	BUNBURY	175	4
	GERALDTON	F 369	5
	KALGOORLIE	F 539	4
	ALBANY	413	6
	PORT HEDLAND	F 1308	3
	MANDURAH	74	4
	KARRATHA	F 1247	3
	ESPERANCE	F 650	2
	NEWMAN	F 1017	1
	CARNARVON	F 815	2
	BROOME	F 1675	2
	MERRIDEN	261	3
	TOM PRICE	F 1034	1
	DERBY	F 1792	3
	KUNUNURRA	F 2211	1

F = Flying distance

Fig. 2.2. Population and staff numbers in major country towns.

The programme for a visit is arranged in advance with the senior physiotherapist. This may include tuition on a specific topic, assessment of patients and an overview of the department in action. Visits to isolated communities and appraisal studies of outlying areas in need of a physiotherapy service are also undertaken.

Contacts with the hospital administrator to discuss service provision, equipment and staffing levels are also important. Meetings with the director of nursing services and other members of staff are of value when re-structuring obstetric services.

Clinical discussions with local general practitioners and specialists are leading to greater understanding of the physiotherapist's role in obstetrics and gynaecology, more accurate and quicker referral practices and increased benefit to patients.

Visits to staff in country areas are also supportive in nature, giving encouragement in local problem solving, the maintenance of professional contact and a sounding board for new ideas.

GROUPS WITH SPECIAL NEEDS

Some women in Western Australia are disadvantaged by:
— Their isolation
— The demands of rural industries
— Language or cultural barriers.

Since the co-ordinated service for obstetrics and gynaecology has been established in the State, the special needs of women who are unable to have access to this service continue to be examined. It will take some time to establish and publicise specific programmes for these women. The co-operation of local medical and nursing staff is of crucial importance in this task.

Isolated communities

An example of women living in close proximity to others but in an isolated situation is the female population of Koolan Island. The island is 130 km north of the regional centre, Derby, in the far north of Western Australia. Normal access to Derby from Koolan is via a 40 minute flight and this makes regular attendance at ante and postnatal groups impossible.

Therefore two day 'crash courses' for childbirth preparation and postnatal care are being held on the island four times a year by the Derby physiotherapist and a midwife. This gives women basic knowledge and skills to allow them to practise at home and contact the physiotherapist in Derby for individual advice when necessary.

Isolated women

Pregnant women can be isolated from their peers on cattle stations, large farms and in small communities. They are generally delivered in the nearest large town or in Perth; this involves infrequent antenatal check visits to that town and residence there for the last two weeks of pregnancy. In the interim periods the nearest child health sister (who has a midwifery certificate) or doctor continues the antenatal care.

In the past these women have had no contact with a physiotherapist during their pregnancy and only briefly in the short postpartum period in hospital. Apart from missing any chance of learning physical coping skills for labour, they received no information about back care for any aspect of their lives.

Many of them lead a hard and strenuous life and they need strong abdominal and pelvic floor muscles; they also require instruction in prophylactic care of their backs in relation to their activities with the baby and everyday life.

A physiotherapy education and preparation package is being used to improve this situation. It will originate from the physiotherapy department in the town where the women are being delivered. Ideally the newly pregnant woman will collect the package and receive basic instruction from the physiotherapist on her 'booking visit' to the obstetrician. Future contact is encouraged during each antenatal check visit.

The package contains a cassette with instruction on 'coping with tension for labour and life by relaxation and breathing awareness' on one side. The reverse side applies these skills to labour and is a 'labour practice' session. There is also written material to accompany the cassette.

Finally a booklet 'Book of the Child' is included. It spans the period pregnancy to five years, and has contributions from all the relevant professions including physiotherapy.

The demands of rural industries

In country areas of a sparsely populated large state like Western Australia women are often an important element in the rural labour force. This work will generally take priority over their need to join ante and postnatal groups. Long distances between towns preclude frequent visits by these women.

Banana plantations, citrus and soft fruit orchards, vineyards, growing cereals, running sheep and cattle and market gardens are a few examples of the variety of rural industries.

The times of peak activity when the family give all their energy and attention will vary regionally throughout the State during the year.

Antenatal 'crash courses' carefully timed to avoid peak activities seem the best way of offering a service to rural women. The physiotherapists hold several one-day courses a year in a central location so that women can spend the whole day with their peers gaining basic knowledge and skills. Supporting material in the form of hand-outs allows for continued practice at home and provides information on whom to contact if further advice is required.

Language or cultural barriers

The diversity of language and cultural expectations relating to childbearing make it difficult for some women to have access to services offered by physiotherapists.

Work has commenced with Vietnamese health workers to translate simplified antenatal information relating to back care, preparation for labour and postnatal care. Gradually other ethnic groups are being involved. The physiotherapist has to overcome language or cultural barriers to offer effective care in the sensitive issues related to childbearing.

INTER-PROFESSIONAL LIAISON

Nurses

The WA branch of the Australian College of Midwives and the WA Special Interest Group in Obstetrics and Gynaecology of the APA have formed a 'Combined antenatal education committee'.

Their aim is to foster good working relations and understanding between the two groups, share a weekend annual seminar and set standards of practice for both groups in antenatal education.

A team of nurses and physiotherapists who work with people who are incontinent has started the 'Promotion of Continence Association'. It is to be multidisciplinary in its membership and aims to improve knowledge and practice in all aspects of the treatment and prevention of incontinence.

Doctors

Local and regional clinical meetings with medical staff have already been mentioned. The Special Interest Group in Obstetrics and Gynaecology is seeking closer ties with the Royal College of Obstetricians and Gynaecologists, and has shared the platform at an antenatal seminar which members of both disciplines attended.

Antenatal programme details

1. Early pregnancy group — 'Earlybird'

This group is only possible if there is early notification of pregnancy by the obstetrician or GP. It is known that significant backache in pregnancy can be reduced if 'back school' type of advice is given before the 20th week of pregnancy (See Ch. 5).

Also included in the programme are:
— Useful resting positions
— Reduction of oedema and varicosities
— Exercising for a healthy pregnancy
— Information about the effect of drugs, smoking and alcohol
— Bookings for Preparation for Childbirth course.

Individual assessment and treatment for identified musculo-skeletal conditions is an important part of the service. A dietician and a midwife will take part in this class as well.

2. Preparation for childbirth — starting at 28–30 weeks

Whenever possible a midwife will share each class with the physiotherapist. Other health professionals or lay support groups may also be involved.

In some venues the physiotherapist will take the class alone and the information on labour and parenting be given by a midwife separately.

The following topics are covered by the physiotherapist:
a. Coping with tension for labour and life using Mitchell Physiological Relaxation
b. Breathing awareness
c. Pelvic floor muscles — facts and practice
d. Application of relaxation and breathing skills to the first stage of labour
e. Partner's role in labour including 'rocking back pressure' to alleviate back pain

f. Effective activity in the second stage of labour
g. Labour rehearsal and tour of labour ward
h. Post delivery — class reunion.

Obstetric fitness details

1. Physiotherapy healthy pregnancy class

This title is carefully chosen to distinguish the class from other 'aerobic' or 'fitness' groups, and to emphasise that it is being conducted by a health professional.

Childbirth is usually one of the most athletic experiences of a woman's life, and parenting is as demanding as a marathon. It would therefore seem prudent to enter this phase of life as physically and mentally fit as possible.

For some women, walking or running their way through pregnancy is sufficient; other women appreciate more formal classes. These commence about the 12th week of pregnancy and continue until the expected date of delivery.

Aims of the groups:
a. To provide a feeling of well-being through fitness
b. To encourage a balance between sensible eating, careful exercise and extra rest
c. To foster peer group support
d. To provide information about preparation for childbirth programmes.

Pregnancy changes which affect exercise performance:
a. Uterine enlargement
   — discomfort
   — alteration in posture and centre of gravity
   — supine hypotension
   — fainting
b. Structural changes
   — altered conformation of spine and pelvis
   — diastasis of the abdominal rectii
   — diastasis of the symphysis pubis
   — sacro-iliac joint dysfunction
c. Cardiovascular system
   — 40–50% increase in blood volume
   — decreased resistance in peripheral blood vessels resulting in a heating effect
d. Respiratory system
   — increase in chest size and capacity

— increased respiratory rate
— pressure on the diaphragm
e. Fluid balance
— peripheral oedema due to fluid retention
f. Metabolic rate and fat store
— increases
g. Gastro-intestinal tract changes
— possible nausea, gastric reflux and constipation.

Precautions requiring careful questioning:

a. Past obstetric history
— miscarriage
— stillbirth
— premature labour
— shirodkar suture
b. Changes in blood pressure
c. Bleeding in this pregnancy
d. Medical conditions, e.g. diabetes
e. Pain.

Class format

Before start:
— assess new members
— emphasise that it is a non-competitive group
— members to rest when necessary, not to push through pain or fatigue
— demonstrate how to find pulse and calculate maximum heart rate (MHR 220 minus age).

Action

a. Warm-up — five minutes rhythmic movements
b. Stretch   — five minutes gentle stretching
c. Aerobic   — ten minutes 'keep those feet moving', aim to achieve 60–70% MHR
d. Floor   — slow rhythmic movements using a variety of positions singly and in pairs
e. Specific exercises
— pelvic floor contractions

— abdominal exercises
— pelvic tilting
f. Cool down — gentle stretches in standing, kneeling, sitting
       and lying down
g. Relaxation — Mitchell Physiological Method.

Activities to avoid

— Star jumps and continuous bouncing which stretch the pelvic
   floor and often result in leakage of urine
— Sit-ups with straight legs
— Double straight leg lifting
— Hip abduction in four point kneeling
— Consistently increasing lumbar lordosis
— Overheating.

Group discussions

Allowing time for questions is an important part of these classes.
The informality encourages discussion on topics ranging from
insomnia in pregnancy to options in the labour ward.

Conclusion

There is no evidence to show that fitness guarantees easy labour.
But fitness does promote a feeling of well-being and confidence,
which in turn encourages practice in body awareness skills. A fit
person who is able to cope with tension will conserve energy and
combat fatigue in labour and the ensuing parenting.

2. Physiotherapy postnatal classes

In the weeks following delivery women should be encouraged to
join a rehabilitation programme conducted by a physiotherapist.
    These programmes are designed to reduce the long-term effects
of childbearing and promote fitness and a feeling of well-being
which will enable them to cope with their new role as a mother in
addition to their other activities.
    The postnatal groups will therefore be a continuation of the care
given by the physiotherapist to the women in hospital in the days
following delivery.

Aims of the groups

a. To promote a feeling of well-being through fitness
b. To help women adapt to their new role of motherhood
c. To enhance body image
d. To encourage socialisation — it is important for new mothers to leave their homes and meet others in a similar situation, to exchange experiences and foster peer group support
e. To enable women to discuss their problems with the relevant professional staff
f. For the physiotherapist to elicit any physical problems in the group and be prepared to assess and treat these in privacy.

In some health centres a physiotherapist and child health sister arrange to meet newly delivered women and their babies in a group situation. The women may only attend once in the six week period before their postnatal examination with the obstetrician.

Early postnatal class

Suggested content:

a. Discussion and sharing of birth experiences; also other topics, e.g. depression and labile emotions, visitors, joy and worries of motherhood
b. Advice on self-care with the emphasis on adequate rest and diet — to give the mother time to get to know her baby and facilitate bonding
c. Check for diastasis of the abdominal rectii — give advice on support and exercises
d. Stress the importance of the pelvic floor muscles and their restoration to full function
e. Advice on the avoidance of strenuous exercise; give information about postnatal fitness class.

Main postnatal class

Women are encouraged to join this group on completion of their postnatal examination. They bring their baby to the class and remain in the group until the baby is six months old. At this time most women are ready to resume their normal sporting or exercise activities.

Stating a definite date to leave the group ensures a continuous turnover of women and creates space for new members.

It has been found that it is better not to allow siblings to attend with their mothers unless a crèche is available.

Special considerations

If women with any of the following conditions are identified during or after the class, the physiotherapist will assess and treat them individually in the department for as long as the condition persists. Discussion with the patient's general practitioner follows when this is appropriate:

a. Severe weakness of the pelvic floor muscles when the woman is unable to elicit a contraction
b. Diastasis of the abdominal rectii
c. Dyspareunia due to perineal or vaginal scar tissue
d. Mastitis
e. Backache.

Class format

Before start:

a. Assess new members, noting those with abnormal blood pressure, spinal problems or cardiac conditions
b. Check abdominal muscles
c. Advise participants to stop exercise on pain or fatigue
d. Demonstrate how to find pulse and calculate MHR
e. Check the safety of the babies while their mothers are exercising.

Action

The essential components of an exercise group in the form of warm-up, stretching, aerobic exercises working to 60–70% of MHR, floor work and cool down are arranged in a similar manner to the antenatal class. No repetitive bouncing or star jumps are used.

Emphasis is put on strengthening the pelvic floor and the abdominal muscles, and promoting back care, especially in relation to the activities with the baby.

Towards the end of the class a period of Mitchell relaxation is used to enable women to learn to cope with the pressures of parenting. Discussions on lifestyle management are also used.

Relaxation is alternated with tuition in 'baby massage'. Women bring a towel and suitable oil and practise massaging their babies as a form of 'loving touch'. Physiotherapists find this an effective way of encouraging women who are not natural 'touchers' to increase their tactile contact with their baby. In many cases it appears to have a calming effect on mother and baby and to be useful with 'colicky' babies.

Because women are only able to be members of this group until their babies are six months old it is important that they understand and can indentify the conditions which arise as a result of childbearing, and also have enough confidence in the physiotherapist to be able to seek her assistance.

Gynaecology

Opinions vary as to how many weeks postpartum the change from the use of the term obstetric care to gynaecological care occurs. It appears that if the postnatal examination is conducted six weeks after delivery then conditions arising subsequently become gynaecological. During this period the newly delivered women feel ready to join the physiotherapy postnatal classes.

It is noticeable that here in Western Australia as the number of physiotherapists conducting these postnatal exercise classes grows, there is a marked increase in their interest and commitment to the treatment of all types of gynaecological conditions.

Treatments will fall into two categories:

1. Re-education of the pelvic floor muscles for:

— True stress incontinence
— Part of bladder drill
— Vaginal laxity
— Idiopathic anorectal incontinence.

The conditions are likely to have been caused by childbearing and/or constipation and the menopause.

Re-education of the pelvic floor muscles is an economic treatment in terms of the phsiotherapist's and patient's time as it does not require repeated attendance in the physiotherapy department.

This is an important factor in country areas of the State where women may have to travel long distances to reach the hospital or health centre.

2. Electrical treaments to reduce inflammation and pain increase the extensibility of scar tissue and the stimulation of various tissues.

Some of the modalities used are as follows:
— Ultrasound
— Interferential
— Shortwave diathermy
— Faradism.

Dyspareunia due to tight perineal and vaginal scar tissue is frequently identified in postnatal classes. The use of ultrasound and massage is an efficacious method of coping with a condition which has considerable physical and psychological implications.

Hand-out material for patients

Work has begun to compile accurate, simple and well illustrated hand-outs to cover every aspect of these clinical programmes. These will be printed and used throughout the State.

CONTINUING EDUCATION

Continuing education is an important part of all physiotherapists' development and leads to increasing expertise and job satisfaction. Three aspects of continuing education are described here:
— In-service training
— Postgraduate diploma in obstetrics and gynaecology
— Special interest group.

In-service training

Obstetrics

Since January 1985 Health Department physiotherapists have been introduced to the new obstetric programme in the State during an in-service training course lasting two days.

The course is entitled 'Teaching physical skills for the child-bearing year'; by the end of November 1986 four such courses had been held, training about 170 staff. In subsequent years it is estimated that one course a year will be required to maintain a uniform standard in response to staff changes.

Course content

This is aimed at giving accurate background knowledge and teaching practice, using peer comment, of all aspects of the obstetric programmes given in this text. A procedure manual is available in physiotherapy departments giving the resource and reference material necessary to provide an effective service.

Gynaecology

To date, one course has been held in Perth on 'The role of the physiotherapist in gynaecology'.

Staff in country areas are being given instruction regionally or at single hospitals. Individual assessment and treatment sessions with patients, taken by the author with one member of staff observing, has been found to be an ideal way of increasing therapists' clinical skills. The staff member then continues the follow-up treatments with the patient she has observed and soon has the confidence and expertise to offer the full service.

Postgraduate diploma in obstetrics and gynaecology

The School of Physiotherapy at Curtin University of Technology has recently added obstetrics and gynaecology to the other postgraduate diplomas it offers. The four advanced specialisation units for this subject are added to the compulsory health sciences core units to obtain the postgraduate qualification.

Outline of the advanced specialisation units

1. Embryology
   Anatomy, physiology and psychology of reproduction
   Prevention, assessment and treatment of spinal and pelvic
       conditions associated with pregnancy
   Comparative study of methods of relieving tension
   Anatomy and physiology of respiration.
2. Planning and management of obstetric groups
   Processes of labour — normal and abnormal
   Mechanism and control of pain
   Process of breast feeding, bonding and father's role
   Sexuality in the childbearing year
   Psychological effects of parenting, perinatal death and
       bereavement

Postnatal complications in mother and child and their treatment
Skills in neonatal treatment procedures
Skills in inter-professional liaison.

3. Anatomy of urinary tract, micturition and disorders associated with pregnancy
Diagnosis and treatment of incontinence
Promotion of continence
Assessment, treatment and psychology of gynaecological conditions
Sexuality through the life-cycle
Psychosexuality and sexual dysfunction
Counselling education and treatment
Evaluation of treatments and record keeping.

4. Clinical practice — in various settings
   — demonstrating advanced skills in group processes in parent education and professional education
   — skills in individual treatment and counselling for obstetrics, gynaecology and sexual problems
   — advanced ability to maintain records, evaluate treatments and share knowledge.

Special Interest Group in Obstetrics and Gynaecology

This is one of the many special interest groups of the Australian Physiotherapy Association (APA). Each State and Territory has its own group and shares a national group. The latter meets each year at the annual conference of the APA; there is also a national journal published twice a year.

The Western Australian group meets formally five times a year for lectures from specialist speakers covering a wide range of topics associated with obstetrics and gynaecology. The lectures are recorded and sent in cassette form to country members throughout the State.

The meetings also provide a useful platform for discussion and the exchange of new ideas.

THE FUTURE

The role of the physiotherapist in obstetrics and gynaecology is slowly being more clearly defined and understood in the minds of physiotherapists, other health professionals and the public in Western Australia.

As this occurs, physiotherapists will be able to increase the prophylactic advice and care given to childbearing women as well as continuing to expand the postpartum treatments.

Menopausal women are now receiving more attention and assistance. The 'Mid-life and Menopause Group' have recognised the need for a physiotherapist to join their discussion sessions and provide treatment on an individual basis when required.

The evergrowing number of senior citizens in Western Australia are encouraged to join one of the Senior Citizens Healthy Life groups run by Health Department physiotherapists throughout the State. As the rate of urgency, frequency and stress incontinence in this age group is at least 30%, pelvic floor exercises and promotion of continence advice are included in the sessions. The women express satisfaction with this information and wish they had received it earlier in their lives. A study is in process to evaluate the effect of teaching pelvic floor exercises to these groups.

In Australia, women's health is increasingly a topic for the political arena. In September 1985 a conference was held in Adelaide, South Australia to mark the end of the 'Decade of Women'. It was arranged by the Advisor for Women's Health of South Australia as a forum for all views to be expressed and discussed.

Political, sociological and economic strategies were put forward to ensure that women occupy their rightful position in the decision-making processes related to them and their families. Great emphasis was also put on the need to shift the provision of care from being illness-orientated to health-orientated.

The prominence of women's health issues and the commendable emphasis on education and preventative care will accelerate. It complements the initiatives for the co-ordinated service in hand in Western Australia by the physiotherapists working in obstetrics and gynaecology.

Sources of pain in labour

Pain in labour appears to be an age-old phenomenon. During this century a school of thought has developed which deduced that because of the long history of pain associated with childbirth, women are conditioned to expect labour pain. They tense against the anticipation of pain and thereby intensify it. The supposition is that women who do not expect pain will indeed have less pain.

Labour pain has been measured on pain scales such as the McGill Pain Questionnaire, a word-based gauge of pain intensity, and the Visual Analogue Scale, a linear measure of pain (Rosen 1977, Melzack et al 1981, Lawrence 1984). Melzack et al (1981) found that labour pain could be of very high intensity, comparable with the pain of chronic backache, toothache or cancer, though it must be remembered that a single contraction is of limited duration. Hassid (1978) distinguishes between pain threshold where a neurological response occurs and tolerance which invokes an individual reaction. It is important to recognise this distinction. Confusion reigns if it is said of a patient in labour that she has a low pain threshold when what is meant is that she has a low pain tolerance level. Researchers tested the pain threshold of black and white women and found virtually no differences (Winsberg and Greenlick 1975). But it is another matter when tolerance is tested. There are wide differences in behaviour while in pain and this is so for all types of pain (Melzack 1977). The study included in this chapter is a measure of how much labour pain was felt (perceived pain) in contrast with how well it was tolerated.

Anatomical components of labour pain

There are plenty of physical reasons for human labour pain. A baby is a fairly large object which has to be pushed through a narrow but to some extent expansile channel. Evolutionary studies of comparative anatomy have shown that man has doubled his head to body proportion in comparison with the great apes. The pelvis has also been modified because it had to adapt to the upright posture and carry the weight of the trunk. In the all fours position the pelvis hangs from the spine, whereas stronger muscles and ligaments and a more solid bone structure are necessary to maintain an erect position with a low centre of gravity. The resultant S-shaped spine relies heavily on the pelvic floor and lower abdominal musculature to hold the pelvic organs in place, including the gravid uterus.

The Australopithecines, man-like apes, who date from between 5 and 1 million years ago, show evidence of having walked upright and may have been one of the progenitors of modern man. Their brain capacity was a little greater than that of a contemporary chimpanzee but was only a third the size of a modern human brain. The proportion of fetal head to maternal pelvis is a vital factor in the feasibility of vaginal birth. If the fetal head is not flexed to present the smallest possible circumference to the pelvis the mechanism may be unworkable, or only workable after a long period of uterine activity and consequent pain. Some evidence points to Neanderthal man faring even worse, having a large 'acromegalic' head and a relatively rigid fetal cranium. These factors may have led to extinction or to adaptation towards homo sapiens who has a domed forehead containing a more developed brain with bigger frontal lobes and considerable flexibility of the fetal skull.

Data is accumulating on the alteration of pelvic shape in mankind to adapt to upright movements. Electromyographical studies in man and the ape have shown up different stresses which have stimulated bony changes to accommodate to alteration of function. These include a backward extension of the ilium to support a massive buttock muscle which holds the trunk erect while standing and walking, particularly walking uphill. The ape has hardly any buttock development. In order to facilitate birth, female anatomy has favoured a broad basin-shaped pelvis, which means that the thigh bones have to be angled in from the hip joints. Most features of evolution have disadvantages as well as advantages, and the trouble with angled thighs is that the hip joint can dislocate more easily and, in the event of a fall, the femur is more likely to break. However, buttock development is a useful stabiliser of the hip joint in women, and strength in the gluteal region is worth retaining into old age.

An unusual feature of the human female is the contour of the vagina. In primates, the vagina is straight. The human vagina is angled forwards to compensate for the angulation of the pelvis to the lumbar spine. The baby is born round a curve, the curve of Carus (Carus was an eighteenth century German anatomist-obstetrician).

Human young are heavier at birth than the young of big primates, and compared with many other mammals there has been a reduction in the number of young in the uterus. The female human being more often than not delivers the young head first, using the head to expand the birth passages. One of the devices which helps human birth to succeed is moulding of the fetal skull. Moloy (1942) found that fetal heads varied in their malleability. 'Hard' heads moulded only with difficulty, while 'soft' heads with more elastic cranial bones allowed more movement at the suture lines. Heyns (1946) noted excessive moulding in Bantu babies, and also concluded that the mothers had very strong contractions and hence were efficient parturients. In evolving a large head and increasing the body weight of the fetus, mankind made genetic adjustments, but the average gestational period did not lengthen (in the chimpanzee it is 8–9 months). There is a tendency for large animals to have long gestational periods (the elephant has 22 months). If the gestational period had become longer for females the mechanical difficulties would have increased. Although there has been some change in body size, this is variable, human beings differing greatly even in one continent. Body size affects pelvis size — obstetricians look at a woman's hands and feet and check her height.

Steer (1975) classified 14 different pelvic types: 4 pure types and 10 with mixed characteristics, the mixed types being more common. Steer gives a 40% incidence of anthropoid pelvis among negro women in the original study. The anthropoid type with the long axis from front to back means that there may be no rotation of the fetal head. It has been observed that Australian aboriginal women had a long thin sacrum (an anthropoid characteristic) and a vestigial coccyx. Their babies had lower than average birth weight (Cox 1981). Late engagement of the fetal head in the pelvic brim was observed by Briggs (1981), who advised careful evaluation before Caesarean section because of the likelihood of a vaginal delivery after a slightly longer than average first stage. In the white (Caucasian) races the gynaecoid pelvis predominates, the transverse being the longer diameter. Llewellyn Jones (1969) states that the Asian pelvis is similar to the Caucasian though smaller, and Zacharin (1980) found the Chinese levator ani to be of 'excellent quality': thick musculature with strong attachments to the pelvis. A strong well-slung pelvic floor may assist rotation of the fetal head.

The simple anatomy of an obstetrically efficient pelvis has been understood for a very long time. Tiny figurines carved from mammoths' tusks featuring a pregnant abdomen and enormous breasts date from the last Ice Age. Preoccupation with birth was reasonable as only by successful birth could the tribe ensure its survival. The figures have wide hips and very angled thighs, suggesting that early man knew about the advantages of a capacious pelvis.

Labour mechanism and its bearing on pain

In medieval times it was believed that the pelvis opened up to admit the child and that the baby actually kicked its way out. Studies by Kapandji (1974) revealed that the opening of the pelvic joints amounts to only a few millimetres of increase in pelvic diameters. The sacro-iliac joint may pivot or slide to produce the movement. From 1–12 mm expansion is said to occur at the pubic symphysis by absorption of fluid, a process known as water imbibition; Russell (1969) produced radiographic evidence that a gravity-aided position with well-flexed hips and knees contributed to expansion of the pelvic outlet. Kapandji described movement at the sacro-iliac joint as a nodding motion (nutation). Counter-nutation brings the coccyx forwards, accentuating the curve of Carus and widening the pelvic inlet. Nutation is the opposite movement, increasing the outlet diameters by taking the sacrum and coccyx backwards. The implication for birth is that this movement should be free to take place. In rare instances, the coccyx is fused to the sacrum and does not move (Oxorn and Foote 1980), but in normal circumstances it will extend at delivery, depending on the flexibility at the sacro-coccygeal joint. Stretching of the perineum may be hampered by a fixed coccyx, for example if the woman is sitting directly on it.

Of Australia in the early nineteenth century, Mary Gilmore writes: 'A woman only had a doctor when she could no longer stand on her feet'. Aboriginal women assisted labouring homestead women on occasion, often with considerable success as their methods were cleaner than those practised by doctors who, not over concerned with asepsis, would wear the same frock coat which might be stiff with blood and pus. Convict women posed a problem with their frequent pregnancies, their infants dying of birth trauma, infection and marasmus. These unfortunate women were collected, particularly in Tasmania, into what were known as female factories, overcrowded dormitories where women lived, gave birth and died. A woman in labour was visited by a midwife known lewdly as a 'fingersmith'. It is probable that women in the last century, when there was little supervision of labour, adopted the position that was most bearable, and if they were not encouraged to recline and relax this may well have been standing and walking about. A medical text in 1816 explicitly states that the parturient should not lie down for long in the first stage: 'it is not expedient . . . . . that she should remain very long at a time in a recumbent posture'. Physiotherapists working towards gravity-aided positions and more mobility in labour should applaud this statement. The new technology of telemetry will give greater freedom when fetal monitoring is necessary.

Positions to expedite delivery have varied according to cultural influences. Some aboriginal women sat in a hole with a step cut in it so that the back was supported to waist level. The hole was lined with leaves. Nearby was another hole with a fire of coals in it: a smoke hole designed to cleanse and seal the perineum. The use of fresh clay, new leaves and ash was a clean way of repairing birth damage. The posture adopted was also mechanically helpful, not unlike the half-sitting position used today. Some tribes squatted over the hole while others sat in a supported position with their feet on a tree trunk, a little like the foot plates or support slings favoured by some hospitals.

Speaking of labour as a whole, Llewellyn Jones (1969) says that the more efficiently the labour mechanism works the less pain there is. A badly working mechanism may mean more hours in labour and consequently more fatigue. Fatigue blunts the ability to control pain.

Physiological contribution to labour pain

It is generally accepted that there are four main physiological factors responsible for labour pain:
a. Stretching of the cervix
b. Pressure on the sacral plexus
c. Stress on pelvic organs, ligaments and muscles
d. Partial ischaemia of uterine muscle.

The cervix is a very tight structure in the nulliparous. The function of the cervix is to keep the baby in the uterus until such time as it is ready to cope with the outside world. Dilatation of the cervix occurs after hormones soften it and power from the uterus overcomes its resistance. This dilatation process is fairly slow, usually occupying about nine-tenths of the whole duration of labour, and in general this is the most painful part. There are exceptions when the cervix opens fast and painlessly and the birth is painful by comparison, perhaps because there has been no time for a build-up of the body's own pain control system to come into operation. Kimball et al (1980) found that women who had a vaginal birth had higher levels of endorphin than those who had a Caesarean section. In the majority of primiparae it has taken some hours for the muscular uterus to overcome cervical resistance so that the presenting part can fit through. The cervix is richly supplied with nerve endings sensitive to pressure and stretch. Impulses are sent constantly to the central nervous system during a contraction where they can be reviewed for their importance, in other words their pain message.

Low back pain is very common in early labour. After that, in many labours the pain becomes more noticeable in the low abdomen which can be put down to referred pain from stretch of the cervix. As this is usually a stronger sensation than pressure on the back, there tends to be a 'busy line' going to the brain from the front, and the painful sensations from the back fail to get into the communication system. However, if pressure on the bony sacrum is very great, as it can be when there is a posterior position of the fetal head, then back pain often predominates. The bundle of nerve fibres constituting the sacral plexus is being periodically squashed, giving rise to multiple signals which can overcome the inhibitory pain mechanism. Another explanation of severe back pain is that it is referred pain from neurones receiving cervical impulses which are closely associated with transmitting centres for the back (Bowsher 1977).

Stretch and pressure on pelvic structures, such as ovaries, tubes, bladder and bowel, may cause discomfort as the head moves well down into the pelvis; occasionally scarring or adhesions appear to be responsible for pain. Ligaments have been subjected to helpful preliminary softening in pregnancy. They must submit to forceful stretching in labour. The force on organs and ligaments is multiplied if the mechanics are only marginally workable; either a big head in a small pelvis or a badly fitting head. Muscle stretch occurs mainly in the second stage when the pelvic floor is dilating.

The uterus is largely muscle tissue, and although its workings are automatic and involuntary, it is able to send messages that its blood supply is under threat and this can lead not only to pain but to danger for the fetus. An ischaemic uterus is short of oxygen. In normal labours it is unlikely that partial ischaemia is a source of pain as the upper two-thirds of the uterus is seldom painful. But if the uterus is contracting tetanically, that is having little or no rest between contractions, pain acts as a warning. In primitive societies the situation can be serious. Eventually the uterus may rupture. An overworking uterus with a mechanical problem may be assisted by epidural anaesthesia which will ensure greater relaxation of internal pelvic musculature and relieve the pain.

Psychological climate for labour pain

Psychological functioning sets the human being apart. Animal pain has been extensively studied, and it is because of research into pain pathways in animals that so much is known about how pain impulses travel. But interpretation of pain is a dividing factor between the human who knows (homo sapiens) and becomes discouraged about the period of pain still to be faced, and the animal that only recognises pain while it is there. Dobzhansky et al (1977) paints a gloomy picture of human labour when he says 'the globular head of the infant with its voluminous brain is barely able to squeeze through.' He states that 'childbirth is agonisingly painful, which is a biological absurdity.' Recently, there has been a tendency for women to be brainwashed towards expecting pain-less contractions if they react 'correctly' and have the 'right' atti-tude. But there is evidence all around us that labour is often a painful process for women of all races and it is counter-productive to minimise or dismiss the existence of pain. In fact, if a woman goes into labour expecting no challenge by pain she is likely to be devastated.

Birth arouses tremendous community interest and appears to have done so since man saw a continuity in his generations. Diffi-culty in childbirth has been recognised from earliest recorded history, much of it being associated with magical processes and superstition. Egyptians had a goddess to look after obstetrical matters, as did the Greeks and the Romans whose every action was overlooked by some deity. Egyptian murals show an obstetric chair with a woman enthroned, giving birth aided by a number of female attendants. The situation is common in historic pictorial art.

It is not known whether women in labour preferred their own sex for reasons of modesty, or that men considered the function of accoucheur demeaning or contaminating. Possibly many factors were involved, but it seems beyond dispute that men were excluded more often than not from witnessing delivery.

Of course there must be many examples in history and pre-history of men taking part in the birth process, either directly or through the couvade, a vicarious sharing of labour pain and sometimes pregnancy ills by the husband who was not necessarily present. Modern involvement of the prospective father is an exciting new development which apparently has never been known on such a scale. This additional assistance, while probably only marginally helpful in assisting labour mechanics, can be of inestimable psychological value.

A study of pain perception and pain reaction in labour

An observational study was performed on nulliparous labour pain in an area with a low epidural rate (14.4% of all births including epidural for Caesarean section) which facilitated the comprehensive assessment of pain. The intention was to assess perceived labour pain in women who had been fully trained by physiotherapists using a standard method of techniques for control of pain, and women who had received no training or minimal training. The perceived pain index was then contrasted with an assessment of pain reaction (Lawrence 1984).

A review of the literature gave the impression that although pain in labour had been researched by many people, including obstetricians, midwives, psychologists, statisticians and physiotherapists, pain was seldom clearly defined or accurately measured. There were problems in obtaining matching groups, in standardising training methods and in taking obstetric events such as epidurals into account.

Pain can be examined in two ways: pain perceived by the patient and pain observed by an onlooker who estimates pain intensity by the patient's behaviour. Because midwives observe labour pain and record their findings consistently, there was no difficulty in devising a scale for observed pain. This parameter was entitled Pain Reaction (PR), and was measured in degrees of patient distress. Perceived pain is less easily measured. For instance, should it be measured at the time of pain, i.e. in labour? Or should the assessment wait until the patient is a few hours postnatal and can think more objectively and comprehensively about her pain? Some researchers found that asking questions in labour distracted the patient, while others waited weeks or months before issuing a questionnaire.

A McGill pain scale was chosen, which had already been successfully used for labour (Melzack et al 1981). To assist in verifying results, a visual analogue scale (VAS) was added to the design. This scale had been found to be accurate for recording labour pain, giving consistent readings over 1–3 days postnatally (Rosen 1977), which suggests that short-term memory of pain is reliable. However, this was checked by doing a re-run of questionnaires for 20 patients on day 5 using a different physiotherapist to issue the second questionnaire. The results confirmed those of Rosen.

The research took place in Hobart, the capital city of Tasmania, which has only two maternity hospitals. By using the venues of all births in Hobart it was possible to do a whole population study, thus avoiding the difficulties involved in randomly allocating women to groups. Matching was done by measuring a large range of explanatory variables for any significant differences between the groups. It was decided that only nulliparous labour pain would be investigated because of the very different conditions that exist, both physically and psychologically, when a woman is having her second or subsequent child.

Method

Over a $4\frac{1}{2}$ month period there were 513 primiparous births in the two maternity hospitals. Elective and early Caesareans before pain had developed were excluded from the sample, as were gestation periods of under 37 weeks, stillbirths and serious medical complications. Questionnaires were given out by ward staff to all primiparae by day 1, to be answered by the end of day 2 (Fig. 3.1). Anyone with a 'late' questionnaire was disqualified. Six physiotherapists with experience of obstetrics collected the questionnaires, making sure all questions were answered. They were also responsible for filling in medical details from the patient's medical record.

The questionnaires consisted of two parts. Part 1 contained questions for the patient on her age, height, occupation, educational standard, fitness before and during pregnancy, her attitude to labour, her pain expectation in retrospect and an evaluation of her

Labour questionnaire.   PLEASE FILL IN PART 1 BY DAY 2.
Part 1.

Age .... Husband/partner-father support in pregnancy .... (yes/no) ..... In labour ......
Height .... (yours) .... (your husband's)
Occupation .... (yours) .... (your husband's)
Education .... (yours) .... (your husband's)
(1. x years High School, 2. Finished H.S., 3. University.)
Fitness .... (before becoming pregnant) .... (during pregnancy)
(1. Competitive sport, 2. Recreational, 3. No sport).
Did you attend 4 or more physio classes in pregnancy? .... (yes/no)
Prospective Birth Attitude ....
(1. Confident, 2. Not sure what to expect, 3. Worried.)
Pain Expectation ....
(1. Pain less than expected, 2. As expected, 3. Greater).
Pain Perceived (Try to list 1 pain word from each group for the 4 parts of labour — e.g. for 1st
Stage you might have A3 B4 C5. If no word in a group applies put 0 for that group).

A	B	C
1. Pinching (Grabbing)	Mild	Annoying
2. Pressing (Stretching)	Discomforting	Troublesome
3. Gnawing (Stinging)	Distressing	Miserable
4. Cramping	Horrible	Intense
5. Crushing	Excruciating	Unbearable

1st Stage .... Transition ....
2nd Stage .... Birth ....
Mark with a cross on the line the most intense degree of pain in entire labour.
Mild pain ————————————————————————————— Intolerable pain

Part 2.
Weight of baby .... Head circ .... Apgar ....
Length of labour
1st St (Dilation) .... 2nd St ....
Station of Head/Hrs to delivery .... 1. Engaged, 2. At brim, 3. Not engaged
State of membranes ....
(Spontaneous rupture (S), ARM, ARM (D) — during labour)
Drip .... Syntocinon induction (I) augmentation (A) Plain Drip (P)
Analgesia .... (1. None, 2. NO₂ only, 3. Pethidine — up to 100 mg,
4. Pethidine — over 100 mg, 5. Morphine, 6. Epidural, 7. G.A.
Pain reaction ....
(1. Very calm, 2. Calm, 3. Slightly distressed, 4. Distressed, 5. Very distressed.)
Type of delivery ....
(1. Normal, 2. Low forceps, 3. Mid forceps, 4. Ventouse, 5. C/S.)
Obstetrician ....
Position ....

Fig. 3.1 Labour questionnaire.

actual pain. The height, occupation and educational standard of the father was also requested, and whether he was there to support the patient in labour.

In the pain section patients had to choose words describing pain for 4 different phases of labour: first stage, 'transition', second stage, and birth. These pain words came from the McGill Pain

Questionnaire (Melzack 1975), adapted to suit labour. The resultant score was called the Pain Rating Index (PRI). Scoring was averaged so that a patient with a labour that culminated in a Caesarean section or an epidural which deleted pain in one, two or three of the phases, could still be compared with a patient who had undergone all four phases.

The Visual Analogue Scale (VAS), a 10 cm line which was marked 'mild pain' at one end and 'intolerable pain' at the other, was used to record the intensity of the worst pain in labour. This could occur in any of the four phases.

Part 2 recorded medical information such as duration of the first and second stages, the state of the membranes, whether an induction or augmentation was performed, the amount and type of analgesia, the position of the fetal presenting part, the mode of delivery and the obstetrician responsible for the patient. Neonatal details comprised weight, head circumference and Apgar score. The pain reaction score (PR) was also included in Part 2.

After the medical exclusions and disqualifications for late or inadequate questionnaires were subtracted from the 513 possible candidates, the sample consisted of 338 primiparae whose nulliparous labour was to be investigated. Two-thirds of the sample (228) received prenatal training. Training consisted of a minimum of four classes taken by experienced physiotherapists who were all teaching the same techniques. Those who dropped out in the early stages before techniques had been fully grasped were designated 'untrained'. The method used was the psychophysical approach described by Williams and Booth (1985).

In this study the patient was 'blind' for the period under study — i.e. labour. Midwives and obstetricians also were not told that the experiment was taking place. Special measures were taken to prevent bias among the physiotherapist assessors. A set of rules was given out on how patients were to be approached, how pain questions were to be answered and how to interpret the medical records consistently. Pain scores from all questionnaires were averaged for each assessor in order to check consistency. There proved to be very little difference between the averages, which meant that no matter which physiotherapist did the assessing the result was the same.

The method was chosen to interfere as little as possible with normal labour ward procedures, bearing in mind the advice of Huntingford (1965) that anyone who knows they are taking part in an experiment is liable to alteration in behaviour.

Results

The data was fed into a computer and analysed using analysis of
variance (Table 3.1). Pain perceived by the patient was found to
be positively related to six variables: duration of the first stage of
labour, analgesia level, mode of delivery, pain expectation and pain
reaction ($p<0.01$). Fetal position was positively related to perceived
pain but the result was less conclusive ($p<0.05$). The patient's

Table 3.1 The relation between measures of pain and explanatory variables.
Results from application of analysis of variance

Explanatory variable	PRI		VAS		PR	
	R²	Prob.	R²	Prob.	R²	Prob.
Physiotherapy training	1	n	0	n	7	★★
Analgesia	8	★★	0	n	20	★★
Pain reaction	6	★★	4	★★		
Delivery	8	★★	3	n	3	★
Mother's education	0	n	0	n	2	n
Father's education	1	n	1	n	2	n
Husband's support	0	n	0	n	0	n
Pre-pregnancy fitness	0	n	0	n	1	n
Pregnancy fitness	1	n	1	n	1	n
Station of head	3	★	1	n	2	★
State of membranes	0	n	0	n	1	n
Prospective birth attitude	0	n	1	n	2	★
Mother's occupation	0	n	0	n	2	★
Father's occupation	0	n	0	n	2	n
Infusion	1	n	0	n	2	n
Apgar	4	n	3	n	2	n
Pain expectation	8	★★	21	★★	2	★
Age	0	n	0	n	1	n
Height	2	n	0	n	1	n
Difference in heights	3	★	0	n	0	n
Head to height ratio	1	n	0	n	1	n
Weight	0	n	0	n	0	n
Duration 1st stage	6	★★	4	★★	7	★★
Duration 2nd stage	1	n	1	n	0	n
Duration total	6	★★	4	★★	6	★★
Obstetrician	5	n	5	n	2	n
++Position	3	★	1	n	2	n

Notes

1. R² is the proportion of variation in the response variable (i.e. either PRI or VAS or PR) which can be
related to variation in the explanatory variable.
2. 'Prob.' provides an assessment as to whether the relation between response variable and explanatory
variable observed in the sample is likely to be a real effect or merely the consequence of sampling
variation. The symbols used in the table can be interpreted as follows:
'n'   — results consistent with assumption of no relationship
'★'   — weak evidence that variation in response variable is connected with variation in explanatory
variable ($p<0.05$)
'★★'   — strong evidence that variation in response variable is connected with variation in explanatory
variable ($p<0.01$)
++ In the case of Position $p<0.05$ was considered significant because of the demonstrated difference
between the groups and because the percentages of patients in each category was equal between the groups.

reaction to pain (PR) proved to be related positively to duration of first stage, analgesia and physiotherapy training (p<0.01).

Further analysis by least significant difference and chi-squared tests revealed differences between the trained and untrained groups. The trained group had higher perceived pain scores (both PRI and VAS) for the same pain reaction score as the untrained (Fig. 3.2). Furthermore the trained group needed lower levels of analgesia for the same perceived pain levels as the untrained (p<0.01) (Fig. 3.3). Fetal position proved significant in that trained patients did not report higher perceived pain for less desirable positions, namely transverse and posterior positions of the fetal head persisting until second stage, whereas the untrained group did record higher scores for these positions (p<0.05) (Fig. 3.4).

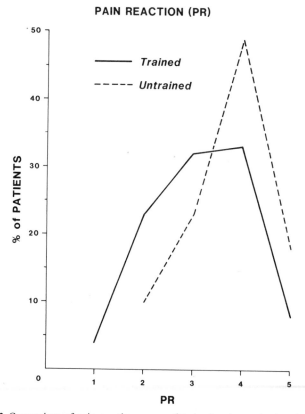

PAIN REACTION (PR)

Fig. 3.2 Comparison of pain reaction scores of trained and untrained patients. 60% of trained patients were given a PR of 3 or lower. Only 33% of untrained patients were rated 3 or lower.

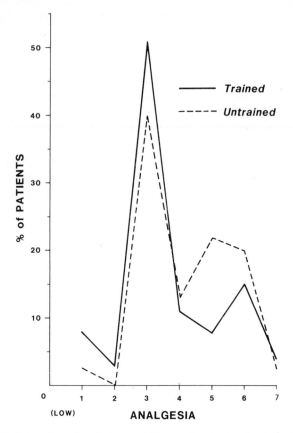

Fig. 3.3 Comparison of analgesic requirements of trained and untrained patients. Trained patients are more strongly represented in analgesic catagories 1–3 (no analgesic, NO_2 only, up to 100 mg pethidine) than untrained patients.

Besides this, spontaneous rotation occurred in a higher number of occasions when the patient had been trained.

In effect, prenatal training enabled women to maintain better control of their labour, although their perceived pain levels were as high as those who had not trained. This was so, regardless of which hospital they went to and also regardless of whether they were public or private patients. Public patients were to some extent disadvantaged by lack of support from the husband or partner–father (there was a greater proportion of single mothers in this group). However, public patients as a group obtained results

PAIN PERCEIVED (PRI)

compared with POSITION

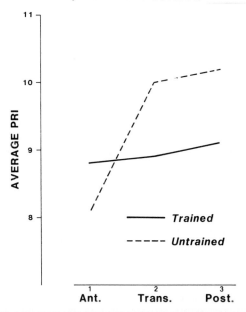

Fig. 3.4 Comparison of average pain rating index for trained and untrained patients with different fetal head positions prior to birth. The rise in PRI for untrained patients with transverse or posterior position is not apparent for trained patients. The percentages of patients in each category were approximately equal between the groups.

equal to private patients if they had attended classes, even if there had been no 'support person' with them in labour.

The relationship of 'pain expectation' to pain showed no differences between the groups. Pain expectation was a measure of how closely the actual labour approximated to what had been envisaged. This relationship was demonstrated in perceived pain scores, particularly the visual analogue (VAS). Women who had more pain than they had anticipated tended to give themselves high VAS ratings, whereas if pain was less than expected, VAS scores were quite low. Pain reaction bore a lesser overall relationship to pain expectation. However, PR scores were lower in the trained group when the labour was unduly long (over 10 hours).

Mode of delivery was only related to pain in that the more complicated the delivery, the higher the pain scores. It is, however,

likely that this was a reflexion of the type of labour which culminated in a certain mode of delivery more than the delivery itself,
e.g. a persistent posterior position resulting after some hours in a
Caesarean section.

Discussion

The most conclusive and important results emerging from this
study were that physiotherapy training did lead to better control
of pain and that trained women needed less analgesic aid in labour.
In Hobart, analgesia is given when control of pain by trained techniques or will power begins to be less effective, so that the two are
interrelated. Several research groups have found that training
reduces the need for analgesia (Furler et al 1964, Sharley 1970,
Huttel et al 1972, Zax et al 1975, Hughey et al 1978).

Duration of labour appears to be closely linked with pain in the
first stage, which is understandable as this is usually the period of
greatest pain. Training appears to increase pain tolerance to some
extent when the first stage is longer than average, possibly because
effective relaxation reduces the fatigue factor. Second stage was
expedited by the obstetrician if necessary, using local anaesthesia
to make the procedure as comfortable as possible. Patients estimated their perceived pain for second stage (both PRI and, where
it applied, VAS), but pain reaction was not recorded by midwives
as a routine. However, according to the PRI scores for the second
stage it would appear that few women found this stage more painful
than first stage. It was noted that the PRI score for the actual birth
was quite often nil (0), and this was an expression of relief from
pain, probably due either to natural numbing of the perineum or
local anaesthesia.

It is interesting that pain expectation was not strongly related to
behaviour in labour in either group. This result suggests that all
women make an effort to control behaviour to their physical and/or
psychological limit, no matter what they expect. An explanation
could be the context of labour pain; Reading (1979) has said that
the context of pain is very important and labour usually has a very
encouraging context. A further inference is that the actual experience of labour overshadows any prior conceptions. It could be
argued that if this is so, why were physical factors such as fetal
birth weight and head circumference and maternal height found to
be unrelated to pain? The author's conclusion is that these factors
were indirectly related to pain under the parameter 'duration',

which would account for cervical dystocia, deflexed head or any problems of feto-pelvic disproportion. Gross disproportion necessitating elective or early Caesarean section was not represented in the study because there was no labour pain to measure. These omissions could have caused some distortion of the results for physical parameters.

There was some evidence that physiotherapy training was instrumental in converting transverse and posterior positions to anterior, but more research will need to be done before these results can be considered entirely conclusive.

The study confirms that prenatal physiotherapy is valuable, and the psychophysical techniques taught are effective for dealing with intermittent pain. Rhythm techniques such as rocking and shallow breathing could enhance endorphin production and large fibre nerve conduction (Lawrence 1982). Ambulation and mechanically advantageous positioning may be helpful in rotating the fetal head. Even if the reduced need for analgesia were the only benefit of training, it would be worth while for the well-being of the newborn and for the mother's conscious awareness and satisfaction.

The experimental material was taken from an unpublished thesis for a fellowship awarded by the Australian College of Physiotherapists. Supervisory advice on the research was obtained from Professor J. F. Correy, Professor of Obstetrics and Gynaecology, University of Tasmania. Mr G. McPherson, University of Tasmania Mathematics Department, computed the results and analysed the statistical data.

REFERENCES

Bowsher D 1977 Central nervous mechanisms and uterine sensation. In: Philipp E E, Barnes J, Newton M (eds) Scientific foundations of obstetrics & gynaecology. Heinemann, Chicago, p 606

Briggs N D 1981 Engagement of the fetal head in the negro primigravida. British Journal of Obstetrics and Gynaecology 88:1086

Cox J W 1981 The antenatal and perinatal characteristics of socio-economically depressed Caucasians. Australian and New Zealand Journal of Obstetrics and Gynaecology 21:20

Dobzhansky T, Ayala F J, Stebbins G L, Valentine J W 1977 Evolution. W H Freeman, San Francisco, p 443

Furler I K, Shield B, Poidevin L O S 1964 Prophylactic preparation for childbirth. Medical Journal of Australia 1:986

Hassid P 1978 Textbook for childbirth educators. Harper and Row, New York, p 19

Heyns O S 1946 The superiority of the South African Negro or Bantu as a parturient. Journal of Obstetrics and Gynaecology of the British Empire 53:405

Hughey M J, Muelin T W, Young T 1978 Maternal and fetal outcome of Lamaze-prepared patients. Obstetrics and Gynaecology 51:643

Huntingford P 1965 Objective results of training on labour. Paper at Obstetric Association of Chartered Physiotherapists

Huttel F A, Mitchell I, Fischer W M, Meyer A E 1972 A quantitative evaluation of psychoprophylaxis in childbirth. Journal of Psychosomatic Research 16:81

Kapandji I A 1974 The physiology of the joints. Churchill Livingstone, Edinburgh, p 68

Kimball C D, Chang C M, Huang S M et al 1980 Immunoreactive endorphin peptides and prolactin in umbilical vein and maternal blood. Paper at Pac Co Obstetrical and Gynaecological Society, USA

Lawrence H 1982 How relevant is antenatal training to pain experienced in labour? Australian Physiotherapy Association National Obstetrics and Gynaecology Group Journal 1: 4: 27

Lawrence H 1984 A study of the effect of antenatal physiotherapy coaching on labour pain in the nullipara. Unpublished thesis

Llewellyn Jones D 1969 Fundamentals of obstetrics and gynaecology. Faber and Faber, London, p 313

Melzack R 1975 The McGill pain questionnaire; major properties and scoring methods. Pain 1:277

Melzack R 1977 The puzzle of pain. Penguin Books, London, p 25

Melzack R, Taenzer P, Feldman P, Kinch R A 1981 Labour is still painful after prepared childbirth training. Canadian Medical Association Journal 125:357

Moloy H C 1942 Studies on head molding during labor. American Journal of Obstetrics and Gynecology 44:762

Oxorn H, Foote W R 1980 Human labor and birth. Appleton-Century-Crofts, New York, p 3

Reading A E 1979 The short term effects of psychological preparation for surgery. Social Science & Medicine 13A (6): 641

Rosen M 1977 The measurement of pain. In: Harcus A W, Smith R B, Whittle B A (eds) Pain — new perspectives in measurement and management. Churchill Livingstone, Edinburgh, p 13

Russell J G B 1969 Moulding of the pelvic outlet. Journal of Obstetrics and Gynaecology of the British Commonwealth 76:817

Sharley C 1970 The value of physiotherapy in obstetrics. Australian Medical Journal 1:1159

Steer C M 1975 Moloy's evaluation of the pelvis in obstetrics. Plenum Medical Book Company, New York, p 10

Williams M, Booth D 1985 Antenatal education — guidelines for teachers, 3rd edn. Churchill Livingstone, Edinburgh

Winsberg B, Greenlick M 1975 Pain response in negro and white obstetrical patients. In: Weisenberg M (ed) Pain — clinical and experimental perspectives. C V Mobsby, St Louis, p 158

Zacharin R F 1980 Pulsion enterocele: review of functional anatomy of the pelvic floor. Journal of the American College of Obstetricians and Gynecologists 55: 2: 135

Zax M, Sameroff A J, Farnum J E 1975 Childbirth education, maternal attitudes and delivery. American Journal of Obstetrics and Gynecology 123:185

Maternal effort during labour and delivery

INTRODUCTION

Changing practice in the place and mode of delivery has impinged upon a woman's freedom during the process of labour. As well as the increase in medical intervention, control of her activity during labour and birth can also be seen as a form of intervention. During this century, the management of labour and delivery in hospitals has involved unnatural positions, controlled breathing, and forced pushing. While such interventions may have been well intentioned, scientific studies have since shown that normal physiology is disturbed. Psychologically, the woman is hard pressed to perform and, philosophically, this approach runs counter to the latest insights into energy medicine or human physics.

The word labour is still used in association with childbirth. We have been told of 'Childbirth without Pain', and 'Childbirth without Effort'. Labour denotes hard work and can involve fear and pain. We have adopted techniques for distraction and disassociation to control labour. The goal of childbirth education and labour coaching has been to stay on top of the situation. Mothers are taught to shut out internal stimuli and make every effort not to give in or lose control. Rehearsed, resolute and goal-orientated, many couples go into labour as into combat. It has been found that effort and resistance increase if the mother tries to control the dynamics of birth. Unnecessary muscle work reduces awareness, greater exertion is required to accomplish the result and a vicious circle develops. Childbirth films tend to reinforce the expectation that birth involves tremendous physical output. The woman is shown panting and straining, cheered on by those around her as she labours, often flat on her back. Many birth films, particularly in the United States, are instructive rather than enlightening, endorsing a particular teaching method, and failing to convey the essence of the birth experience. One notable exception is the film *Birth in the Squatting Position*, made by Drs Moyses and Claudio Paciornik in Curitiba, Brazil. Several selected births show the almost effortless descent and rotation of the baby without any outside assistance other than gravity.

MATERNAL POSITION

Maternal position has a direct influence on the length of labour, maternal effort and the level of pain experienced. The supine position for delivery (conspicuous in its absence among non-industrialised cultures, according to anthropologists), came into vogue in France when Louis XIV wanted to watch his own child being born. Despite the number of studies showing the benefits of the upright position and ambulation during labour, in many hospitals women continue to be placed supine, not only in the United States but all over the world. The routine use of fetal monitoring and/or an intravenous drip serves to confine a woman to bed, mostly on her back. This position puts a strain on the circulatory system as major blood vessels are compressed. Supine hypotension caused by low cardiac output may result, and the blood supply to the fetus may be diminished. Contractions are less efficient in supine and the woman labours longer. Worse may be to come in second stage if she remains flat. Then she must exert herself without gravity to help and actually push the baby uphill through the pelvic outlet. In addition, her legs are sometimes confined in stirrups; this uncomfortable position has been associated with subsquent lower back pain or sacro-iliac strain, especially if the hips are not positioned symmetrically.

Many researchers, such as Caldeyro-Barcia (1978), Dunn (1976), Newton et al (1960) and Humphrey et al (1974), have shown that labour is more physiological, and contractions are most efficient, when the woman works with gravity instead of being mechanically disadvantaged in the supine position. Caldeyro-Barcia found improvement even with the trunk at an angle of only 40 degrees to the horizontal. He observed a significant association between the supine position and forceps delivery. The vertical position did not increase moulding of the fetal head, nor does squatting lead to a perineal explosion as has been feared by some obstetricians. The drive angle of the uterus relates to the angle formed by the axis of the maternal and fetal spines. Ideally this angle is between 60 and 80 degrees, which is naturally accomplished in standing or squatting. At this angle, contractions drive the fetal head posteriorly to facilitate its descent around the curve of Carus. If the woman is lying flat, the angle is decreased, causing contractions to drive the head more anteriorly. Labour is thus less efficient (Gold 1950).

Flynn et al (1978) found that ambulation shortened the duration of labour and decreased the need for analgesics and the incidence of fetal heart abnormalities. Apgar scores were greater in the ambulant group; more patients in the recumbent group required augmentation with oxytocic drugs. Ehrstrom, who designed a Swedish birth chair, discovered from X-rays of the pelvis that the outlet was increased up to 1.5 cm in a sitting position. Michel Odent (1979) estimates that the supported squatting position adds 15% to the expulsive force.

J. G. B. Russell (1969) has done some interesting work on maternal positions for delivery. He suggests that one-third of women in the world deliver without the possibility of medical aid and in these circumstances they have found for themselves the most advantageous position — upright. In the non-pregnant woman Russell found by radiological examination an increase in the pelvic outlet of up to 28% in the squatting as opposed to the supine position. (Presumably the movements of the pelvic joints are even greater in pregnancy due to ligamentous laxity.) Obstetricians conscious of this, will require a woman to try squatting before doing a forceps delivery for delay in the second stage (assuming the fetus to be uncompromised).

CONTROLLED RESPIRATION

Breathing is an activity that can be both conscious and unconscious. Normally, we never think about this essential life-giving activity, as the body automatically adjusts the rate or depth. Despite this natural efficiency, couples may be taught through childbirth education to adopt artificial breathing patterns. Women may be encouraged to change breathing levels as labour contractions become more intense. This control of breathing by contrived techniques is taught primarily for distraction. Exertive breathing may possibly be helpful in a short labour, but the gaseous exchange can become unbalanced if labour is prolonged. The women who exclaim, 'I could never have gone through labour without the breathing', are, in my experience, just the ones who could. Others, when the effort involved in an artificial pattern of respiration becomes more than they can manage, feel that they have failed. It is difficult to understand the justification for altering something as fundamental as normal breathing, especially during the increased metabolic demands of labour. Recipes for paced respiration rarely take individual variation into account. In pregnancy, many physiological adjustments have occurred in the cardiovascular, musculoskeletal, and respiratory systems. Alveolar ventilation, tidal volume, cardiac output, and blood volume are increased, to give just a few examples. The whole system is perfectly designed so that maternal and fetal blood gases are adequately exchanged. It would seem preferable to study the effects of spontaneous breathing in labour before deciding to alter it, but, like technological interventions, usage has validated acceptance prior to a thorough investigation of the benefits and hazards. The few studies that have examined breath control for pain dealt not with childbirth, but electric shocks. The results are conflicting, and breathing patterns are compared with one another without using normal breathing as a control.

There is an enormous range in individual respiratory rate. This personal feature of breathing is naturally regulated depending on position, activity, emotional state, metabolism, room temperature, and many other factors. The average respiratory rate is 16 breaths per minute, but the range is between 10 and 25 per minute. This point is brought home clearly when a group of expectant couples count their individual breathing rate for one minute. During a preparatory class couples should be given the opportunity to make their choice on the basis of experience, feeling the difference. For example, ask them to quietly observe their breathing rhythm, without attempting to control it in any way, simply being quiet and passive as if they were 'being breathed', just allowing the air to flow in and out. The next stage is to perform slow, deep breathing, typically known as 'Level 1'. The breath is deliberately controlled, and the diaphragm is consciously moved, at a rate of about 10 breaths per minute, which is a 6 second cycle. Then the paced respiration is stopped and the couples return to observation of the normal breathing pattern, tuning into what is happening without doing anything to control it. People are usually surprised to feel the amount of effort required in pacing respiration, even at the slowest level with no likelihood of hyperventilation.

Control of breathing becomes more tiring the longer it is done, and the more complex the technique. Prolonged control of respiration ultimately expends energy, disrupts body rhythms, and diminishes relaxation. If not instructed to breathe according to a certain format, women will adapt their breathing in response to contractions. A woman's breathing provides some clinical information about the stage of her labour, and skilled midwives may not need to do vaginal examination to judge the progress.

SECOND STAGE

In some units, not only are women still made to push longer and harder than is necessary or beneficial, but they may also be forced to do so before the uterus is ready. Ironically, it can happen that the less the desire to push, the harder the woman is encouraged to strain. However, there may be a physiological lull between full dilation and the establishment of the natural expulsive urge, an interval seen more in primipara and that laboratory of alternatives, homebirth. But in hospital it is sometimes unobserved because of the preoccupation with haste and active management.

The expulsive urge begins to be felt when the fetal head descends low enough to stimulate the stretch receptors in the pelvic floor muscles. Stimulation of these proprioceptors leads to increasing levels of endogenous oxytocin, mediated by the posterior pituitary. This neuroendocrine reflex was documented by Ferguson in 1941. Any woman in labour can verify that artificial rupture of the membranes, manual rotation, an enema, or vaginal examination causes subsequent stronger contractions. Breastfeeding to encourage separation of the placenta is another example of this biological phenomenon. Likewise, the proprioceptors in the rectum may be stimulated by pressure from the head, causing a premature urge to push, especially if the woman is lying supine.

Various studies have been made of the relationship between oxytocin levels and uterine activity in the second stage of labour. Goodfellow et al (1983) suggested that epidural anaesthesia, which blocks the pelvic autonomic nerves, abolishes the rise in oxytocin and so affects the contractions. Vasicka (1976) found that any form of local or regional anaesthesia immediately diminished oxytocin output. The diminished oxytocin was thus shown to be a factor in the resultant increased forceps delivery rate. A further factor which may lead to an instrumental delivery is the loss of sensation and the fact that the stretch receptors are no longer stimulated. Women find it difficult to force pushing if there is no guiding urge. Imagine, as you read this, if you were forced to move your bowels in the absence of any desire to do so, and within the next five minutes! Unfortunately, a great many people *do* force bowel movements with excessive effort of accessory muscles. Thus, it is commonly accepted that the straining required for chronic constipation is the best description of how a woman gives birth. The woman can be asked to lift her lower limbs (unless they are confined in stirrups) and her upper trunk against the force of gravity. Even if she is propped, the pulling on her legs tenses her pelvic floor. Excessive straining with the breath held can have severe cardiovascular effects. This forced effort with a closed glottis is known as the Valsalva manoeuvre. It was named after an Italian physician in the seventeenth century who recommended this technique for expelling pus from the middle ear. The danger of the Valsalva manoeuvre during childbirth is that it may be prolonged beyond 5 or 6 seconds, after which disturbance in maternal physiology can occur.

Researchers, led notably by Caldeyro-Barcia, began to examine spontaneous pushing efforts in the late 70s. Pushing, like breathing in labour, had long been directed by others before normal parameters were understood. Caldeyro-Barcia measured the progressive increase in the work done by the uterus and the abdominal muscles — work being the force measured by the amplitude of the contraction and the duration of the effort. For the purposes of analysis, he divided the second stage of labour into three phases. By the final phase, the spontaneous pushing efforts of the mothers had increased threefold. The women in Caldeyro-Barcia's study were not directed when and how to push. They simply pushed according to the varying length and intensity of the urges within contractions, and from contraction to contraction. The average number of pushing efforts per contraction was about 4, with an average duration of only 5 seconds. Average intra-uterine pressure at the peak of the efforts was 88, 107 and 119 mmHg in the first, second and third phases of second stage. The resting interval between each spontaneous effort within the one contraction averaged 2 seconds and facilitated homeostasis. Rest and breathing movements during these intervals minimised the fall in maternal P_{O_2} and rise in P_{CO_2} during the second stage.

Transient Type 1 dips of the fetal heart rate may occur, showing head compression during the expulsive urge, but these fluctuations are benign. No difference in fetal blood values was found between short second stages and those that lasted up to 120 minutes. Nor were there any differences in the Apgar scores. In fact, the average value of the fetal P_{O_2} (27 mmHg in the umbilical artery and 33 mmHg in the umbilical vein) and pH (7.33 and 7.38) were higher than normal values. Caldeyro-Barcia associates forced straining with the need for episiotomy, as there is insufficient time and relaxation for the perineum to distend adequately. Caldeyro-Barcia also undertook research on the effects of the Valsalva manoeuvre during childbirth. Pushing efforts that were directed by an attendant were always longer than those spontaneously expressed by the woman. The amplitude of the effort was over 100 mmHg, and one bearing-down effort, unusually, lasted almost 20 seconds. Maternal blood pressure, measured in the femoral artery, fell to 70/50 mmHg, maternal Po_2 fell to 54 from 104, and fetal Po_2 fell to 21 from 27. The greatly reduced blood flow to the placenta was reflected in the fetal heart tracing. After the end of the contraction, the fetal heart rate, originally about 160 beats/min, fell to between 100 and 130 beats/min, and the drop continued after the end of the contraction. This is considered a prolonged late deceleration, a Type II dip, associated with uteroplacental insufficiency. This may result in fetal hypoxia, acidosis, low Apgar scores and Caesarean section. Clearly, second stage conducted in this manner would be limited to less than two hours because of the stress and strain of prolonged Valsalva manoeuvres.

RECOMMENDATIONS FOR AN ALTERNATIVE APPROACH TO CHILDBIRTH

We have seen that maternal effort is increased by immobility, contrived respiratory techniques, and straining with the breath held. How, then, can this undue exertion be reduced and replaced with physiological alternatives? Much pressure can be taken off the birthing couple if, instead of trying to control the labour, they allow it to take its natural course. Thus reassured women would not have to ask those two questions commonly reported by maternity staff, 'Am I doing it right?' and 'What should I do next?' As well as trying to control the labour, couples are often concerned with their performance — their self-control. If one is concerned with the next step, one automatically tenses toward that future accomplishment. Letting go frees one to experience the present, without regard to the past or future. Yet expectant parents, of course, want resources to deal with pain. I suggest that the pain in labour is the pain of opening up, and a woman's resistance to this is both mental and physical. The cervix and vagina are actively stretched to their limits. Moreover, there are the emotional transitions and psychological regression that accompany the hormonal adaptations in labour, as well as the experience of physical stress.

Additional pain in labour results from tension and fatigue due to exertive coping techniques and insufficient nourishment. What couples need to learn in birth preparation may be difficult to teach. Observing, interpreting and responding to bodily messages is an experience of individual reality that nobody else shares. Yet all the protocols and technological props of labour attempt to create a shared reality. This reality has been paradoxically enforced by childbirth classes. Couples are informed about procedures — when intravenous agents are administered, when the woman will be moved to the delivery room, told to push, and so on. It is generally accepted that much happens beneath the level of the conscious mind including much of birthing. Yet childbirth preparation is frequently set up with lectures, rehearsals and other instruction aimed at the conscious mind. In contrast, in the classes at the Maternal and Child Health Center in Cambridge, USA, we concentrate on partner and group experiences, which not only affirm everybody's individual reality, but where comments or answers can never be judged right or wrong. Preparation for dealing with pain is done at every opportunity. In both couples' classes and exercise sessions, partners sit on the floor with legs astride and feet touching, one leaning backward with extended arms to pull the other forward. This stretches the hamstring muscles to the edge of pain and serves to simulate a contraction as well as providing an excellent stretch to a commonly tight muscle group. Learning to surrender to intense sensations is not as easy as it sounds, for both the mind and the body have to yield. A great deal of physical resistance has mental origins and thus reorganisation within the mind is required.

Labour support, or the lack of it, is another variable. The male partner may be emotionally unavailable during childbirth for many reasons. Thus more couples are bringing along an empathetic, experienced, female support companion, if they have not engaged a midwife. Choice of words is an important part of labour support. Simply asking a mother to bring her baby into the world can turn around a labour, compared with an attendant yelling 'Push, Push, Push'. If a call for emotional help is misinterpreted, this call may result in the clinician requesting the delivery to be accelerated. If fetal well-being can be assured, no woman should have to push before the expulsive urge is well established and actually irresistible. The curve of Friedman's partogram represents an average, and as many women have long labours to the right of the curve as have short labours to the left. The Chinese have a simpler system. According to the *Barefoot Doctor's Manual*, there are just two stages of labour. The first ends with the birth of the baby and the second with the expulsion of the placenta. Our division of labour creates its own added stress, often setting up self-fulfilling prophecies. The extent to which pushing in the second stage can be taught is strictly limited. Vocalisation is preferable to the Valsalva manoeuvre, and the emotional charge that bursts through the inhibitions needs to be respected and affirmed. Sound is a valid expression of accomplishment as well as a physiological response. The effects of the Valsalva manoeuvre on the mechanism of second stage pushing can best be demonstrated by placing the hands on the abdomen during straining with the breath held — the abdominal muscles will be felt to bulge outwards and the pelvic floor muscles to tighten. In contrast, if this is repeated while exhaling with a partially closed glottis an active contraction of the abdominal muscles will be felt and a release of the pelvic floor muscles.

Permitting mothers to birth with ease and dignity can be simple. The key is letting go, the opposite of control. After all, in a normal unmedicated, unanaesthetised birth it is arguable that the uterus knows best. Tension, effort, fight and flight all have their uses in daily life. However, during an uncomplicated birth, the mother can best help by simply allowing it to happen. Learning to let go has benefits reaching beyond the childbearing year. Much therapy today deals with insomnia, sexual dysfunction, anxiety and stress. Interestingly, all these problems share the same common solution — letting go. One cannot master one's response in these situations by control, because of the law of reversed effort. If one tries to fall asleep, tries to have an orgasm, tries to relax, tries to remember the word that is on the tip of the tongue, the effort is self-defeating. Such examples are more appropriate for the birth experience than is constipation, although bowel movements are a biological function that also needs only to be allowed to happen, without forcing. Likewise relaxation cannot be commanded; it happens indirectly as the mind is quietened. Conscious release is not physiologically possible, as there are no nerve endings that convey the state of muscle tension to the cerebral cortex. On the other hand, we are aware of proprioceptors, and so the law of reciprocal relaxation can be invoked to achieve active release, as described by Laura Mitchell. The surrender is a giving in, not a giving up, in order to seek one's own style of birth.

CONCLUSION

Some common cultural approaches to childbirth and the effort and potential hazards involved have been considered. Individually, each may not always be serious, but their adverse effects can be cumulative, especially in the presence of fetal distress. Similarly, Caldeyro-Barcia found that the satisfactory outcome in his studies of spontaneous birth were not related to just one particular modification. The unforced pushing efforts of short duration, avoiding the Valsalva manoeuvre and allowing ventilation of the lungs between pushes, is common sense. Upright positions and spontaneous rupture of the membranes also enhance the natural process. Significantly, the women in his study had no artificial rupture of the membranes, sedatives, analgesics, anaesthesia or oxytocin. It behoves all who are involved with birth to review their philosophy of maternal effort in labour. We need to forget past practices and to avoid clinging to any method. By reducing the effort of our own interventions we will also help make birth safer, easier and more enjoyable for parents.

REFERENCES

Barefoot doctor's manual: A guide to traditional Chinese and modern medicine. Prepared by the Revolutionary Health Care Committee of Hunan Province. Cloudburst Press, Mayne Isle and Seattle

Caldeyro-Barcia R 1979 Physiological and psychological bases for the modern and humanized management of normal labour, presented at the International Year of the Child Commemorative International Congress, Tokyo, Japan 21–22 October

Caldeyro-Barcia R, Giussi G, Storch E, Poseiro J J, Laufaurie N, Kettenhuber K, Ballejo G 1979 The bearing-down efforts and their effects on fetal heart rate, oxygenation and acid base balance. Presented at the 1st International Meeting of Perinatal Medicine June 15–16, Berlin

Caldeyro-Barcia R 1978 The influence of maternal position on labour, and the influence of maternal bearing-down efforts in the second stage of labour on fetal well-being. In: Simkin P, Reinke C (eds) Kaleidoscope of childbearing. Pennypress, Seattle

Dunn P 1976 Obstetric delivery today: for better or for worse? Lancet 1 7963: 790–793

Ehrstrom C 1973 Forlossingstolar Reprint from Recip Reflex (13/72) cited in Kirchoff H 1977 The woman's posture during childbirth, Organorama 14:1, Organon, Oss, The Netherlands

Ferguson J K W 1941 A study of the motility of the intact uterus at term. Surgery in Gynaecology and Obstetrics 73: 359–366

Flynn A M, Kelly J, Hollins G, Lynch P F 1978 Ambulation in labour. British Medical Journal 2: 591–593

Gold E M 1950 'Pelvic drive' in obstetrics: an X ray study of 100 cases. American Journal of Obstetrics & Gynaecology 59(4): 890–896

Goodfellow C F, Hull M G R, Swaab D F, Dogterom J, Buijs R M 1983
    Oxytocin deficiency at delivery with epidural analgesia. British Journal of
    Obstetrics & Gynaecology 90: 214–219
Humphrey M D, Chang A, Wood E C, Morgan S, Hounslow D 1974 A decrease
    in fetal pH during the second stage of labour when conducted in the dorsal
    position. Journal of Obstetrics and Gynaecology of the British Commonwealth
    81:600
Mitchell L 1979 Simple relaxation. Athaneum, New York. John Murray, London
Newton M, Newton N 1960 The propped position for the second stage of labor.
    Obstetrics and Gynaecology 15(1): 28–34
Odent M 1979 Genèse de l'homme ecologique:l'instinct retrouvé. Editions de
    l'Epi, Paris
Russell J G B 1982 The rationale of primitive delivery positions. British Journal
    of Obstetrics & Gynaecology. 89: 712–715
Vasicka A 1976 Lecture at smooth muscle and parturition symposium. Albert
    Einstein College of Medicine. Bronx, N.Y.

Backache in pregnancy

In the survey into backache carried out in 1985 for 'Which', the Consumer's Association Magazine, 28% of the women questioned attributed the start of their backache problems to pregnancy or to gynaecological conditions. It was a similar but subjective impression gained in clinical practice from taking histories of female back pain sufferers, which led earlier to the studies by Mantle et al (1977 and 1981). Obstetricians were, and still are, generally dismissive of complaints of back pain from pregnant women, unless accompanied by obvious signs. Women are told that it is all part of being pregnant, and even to be expected.

The extent of the problem is emerging from evidence in several studies. The first was by Mantle et al (1977) where 48% of a mixed parity, mixed social class, Caucasian group reported troublesome or severe backache at some stage during their recent pregnancy. In a second study by Mantle et al (1981), of a primiparous Caucasian group from a mixture of social classes who received special instruction in back care early in pregnancy, 32% reported troublesome or severe backache. In the control group who had received no special instruction, 54% experienced troublesome or severe backache. Nwuga (1982) examined the situation in an upper class Nigerian group of mixed parity, and found 50% complained of back pain during their recent pregnancy which was anything from mild to severe. It would appear possible therefore that about 50% of all pregnant women experienced some memorable and unpleasant back pain in the course of a pregnancy.

THE CAUSES OF BACK PAIN IN PREGNANCY

Subjective evidence suggests that pregnancy does not protect the woman from suffering from most of the conditions of dis-ease present in her peer group. With regard to back pain, surveys have shown that 20–30% of women in the 15–42 age band could be expected to be suffering from back pain at any one time, and a greater percentage still will have experienced back pain at sometime in the previous year. Consequently, it must always be borne in mind by carers that backache in pregnancy is not necessarily caused by that pregnancy, but may be due to any one of the common or rarer causes — known or as yet unknown — of back pain in this age group.

However, it is thought that three factors associated with pregnancy may render some women more susceptible to or even to cause back pain. These factors are: (a) fatigue, (b) increasing and asymmetrical weight gain, and (c) the effects of the hormones relaxin, oestrogen, progesterone and endogenous cortisols on the actual composition of connective tissue. By the same token, it is conceivable that these same factors may produce changes which, for other women, enable the complex machinery of the spine to function better than when the individual is not pregnant.

a. Fatigue

In the first trimester women commonly experience tiredness and emotional lability. Some have nausea and a few feel thoroughly unwell. The blood plasma volume increases through pregnancy by 30–40% while the cell component does not to the same degree. Consequently the haemoglobin level commonly falls a little — dilution anaemia. This may well contribute to the feeling of tiredness. The nausea, emotional lability and even malaise are attributed to the changed hormonal balance. All these factors can result in fatigue which is reflected in the posture and carriage of the person in sitting, standing and walking. The resultant slack, slumped posture will produce pain by drawing joints into unusual positions, altering load bearing, stretching and straining muscles, ligaments and other soft tissues, and adversely affecting blood flow, leading to the build up of waste metabolites in the tissues. Further, fatigue can adversely affect dynamic body positions and usage at work. This is of particular importance if a pregnant woman is expecting or is expected to continue with a heavy daily workload, both mental and physical. Fatigue also appears to lower the pain tolerance level.

b. Increasing and asymmetrical weight gain

Increasing body weight will result in greater compressive loading and torsional strains on all the spinal components. Women are encouraged to restrict their weight gain to 8–12 kg according to their build, but some experience gains of as much as 20–25 kg. Weight gain alone raises all the forces taken through the spine and lower limbs in all normal postures except lying. It can also change physical anatomical relationships. For example, increased loading could be sufficient to narrow interdiscal spaces, and so the size of intervertebral foramina, to produce nerve root compression in some cases. In other women the extra loading on the sacral prominence may tip it further forward and downward, increasing the lumbar lordosis which in turn may cause over-riding of lumbar facet joints and may place additional strain on the sacro-iliac joints and the ligaments. The weight gain of pregnancy is predominantly anterior (i.e. the abdominal component), occurs chiefly in the third trimester, and necessitates postural adaptations. The protuberant abdomen will cause a woman to fall forwards unless she throws back her shoulders and thus moves the body's centre of gravity backward. This results in a range of possible adaptations from hip and knee flexion, with an increased lumbar lordosis, thoracic kyphosis, cervical extension and with a forward thrusting chin, to 'a sway back' whereby the hips extend and the lumbar spine flexes.

The weight gain and postural adaptation could also put further strain on a damaged disc and therefore be an accumulating cause toward, or the actual precipitating cause of, a disc protrusion. Both weight gain and postural adaptation could also result in facet joints over-riding sufficiently to produce pain and inflammation of capsule and synovium. However, some patients who have experienced back pain pre-pregnancy, apparently due to a disc protrusion, are improved in pregnancy possibly as a result of an increased lumbar lordosis. Pregnancy does provide some positive benefit for the spine. The raised intra-abdominal pressure together with the rising abdominal uterus in the third trimester of a pregnancy may well serve to support and helpfully strut the lumbar spine anteriorly. Pregnant women are less able to bend forward, are less likely to attempt heavy lifting, and tend to avoid lateral flexion because it throws them off balance. All this may have beneficial effects.

Finally, but very importantly, the tenderness, enlargement and increase in weight of breasts can cause changes in posture often quite early in the pregnancy. Some women will round their shoulders and flex their thoracic spine to protect sensitive breasts and even to hide the increase in size. Others will throw their shoulders back to take the extra anterior weight or slump with fatigue later in the day. Further postural adaptations to these changes may be needed and resulting pain can be felt in a number of possible areas.

Unfortunately the assessing physiotherapist rarely has had the advantage of observing and examining the individual prior to the pregnancy, and therefore has nothing but an idealised norm with which to compare and from which to advise a pregnant client or patient.

c. The effects of hormones on connective tissue

The pelvis consists of the two innominates and the sacrum. These three bones articulate at the symphysis pubis and the right and left sacro-iliac joints. Thus a bony ring is formed through which, incidentally, the fetus must pass during the birth process in the case of a vaginal delivery. The pelvis constitutes the bony part of the mechanism by which the main body weight is transferred to the two lower limbs in standing, to one lower limb and then the other in walking, and to the ischial tuberosities in sitting. The three bones are held together by some of the strongest ligaments in the body.

The sacrum supports the weight of the spine and upper trunk, and, by virtue of its wedge shape, is virtually suspended between the innominates by the immensely strong, dense interosseous and posterior sacro-iliac ligaments. Fibres of these ligaments, in the cadaver, detach themselves from their periosteal junctions rather than tear when the bones are forcibly separated (Meckel 1816, Sashin 1930). Loading of the sacrum tenses these ligaments and draws the articular surfaces of the ilia into firmer approximation to the sacrum. This constitutes a locking device, particularly when the congruent irregular surfaces of the two sides of the joint are considered. In addition, the strong sacro-tuberous and sacro-spinous ligaments control forward rotation of the sacrum on the innominates under heavy loading.

The notion that the two sacro-iliac joints and the symphysis pubis were immobile except in the pregnant or very recently parturent woman, or as a result of anomaly or pathology, is now discounted. It is accepted that normally these joints are mobile, and it is only the degree of mobility which usually changes as part of pregnancy, taking up to five months after delivery in some women to return to their pre-pregnancy range.

Regardless of sex, in the average person the range of movement is small, and at its most simplistic seems to consist chiefly of a nodding movement of the sacrum about a transverse axis situated approximately 10 cm below the sacral promontory. Weisl (1955) demonstrated a ventral shift of the sacral promontory of about 5.5 mm when subjects changed from lying to standing. Any ventral movement of the sacral promontory further tenses the interosseous and posterior sacro-iliac ligaments, thus further approximating the ilia to the sacrum. In that the sacrum is wedge-shaped, ventral shift widens the distance between the ilia, as measured by the distance between the posterior superior iliac spines.

However, most pelvises are asymmetrical to a greater or lesser extent in gross structure. Further, the irregularities and undulations of the sacral and iliac surfaces of the joints are highly individual and can vary from left to right within the same person. Also, the general plane of the sacro-iliac joints and the lumbo-sacral facets can be markedly different from side to side, so the axis and range of the resulting movement of the sacrum on the ilia is individual and may vary from left to right. The work of Grieve (1980) shows some interesting correlations between pain and hypermobility, and moots a possible effect by the contraceptive pill in this regard.

Before the hazards of X-rays were appreciated, the changes in pregnancy in the three pelvic joints were well documented. Abramson et al (1934) noticed that relaxation of the symphysis pubis, beginning in the first half of pregnancy, reached a maximum by the last weeks of pregnancy and returned to normal by 5 months postpartum. Sclerosis of the sacro-iliac joints, osteritis condensans ilii, is seen on X-ray after childbirth, indicating transient stress. This usually disappears in a few months to reappear more permanently amongst older women. The normal width of the symphysis pubis of 4 mm increases through pregnancy to about 9 mm, and it is claimed that movement increases by about two and a half times. Any symphyseal movement must be reflected in the sacro-iliac joints but need not be symmetrical. The author has cared for a patient whose symphysis pubis apparently spontaneously separated toward the end of pregnancy and another where this seemed to occur during labour. Hagan (1974) described snapping sounds on vertical symphyseal movement in three patients postpartum. Fraser (1976) reported that 96% of 115 women examined postpartum in standing, supine and prone lying had sacro-iliac torsion. In 75% of these, it was a forward rotation of the right ilium on the sacrum, such that the right anterior superior iliac spine was lying below the level of the left, viewed in standing. However, the findings of Lewit et al (1970) must lead to scepticism that these were all due to pregnancy. Lewit observed pelvic torsion in almost 40% of a group of 450 school children.

It is therefore possible that for some women this joint laxity and resulting additional movement can be painful by virtue of the strains and pressures it places on associated soft tissues surrounding any or all of the pelvic joints. This may be more so where one sacro-iliac joint moves more freely than the other, even over-riding and becoming stuck, causing extra strain around the mobile side or more strain within the joint on the less mobile opposite side. This forward rotation will limit hip flexion on the lower side and, when measured in supine, produce apparent leg lengthening on the affected side by virtue of the altered position of the acetabulum in relation to the other (DonTigny 1985). When measured in sitting the leg on the affected side will appear shortened. Fraser claims a distinctive right left pattern of associated spinal pain of either right sacro-iliac, left dorsal 12, right dorsal 8, left dorsal 2, right cervical 2–3, or of right sacro-iliac, left mid-dorsal, right cervical 2–3.

The laxity is not limited to the joints of the pelvis: all joints are affected to a greater or lesser degree, but to a lesser degree in human to that reported in animals. However, it is of interest that Calguneri et al (1982) showed a significantly higher increase in joint laxity in second pregnancies compared with that in primigravid women, with no further increase in subsequent pregnancies. It is possible that the same increase may pertain to spinal and pelvic joints, for both Mantle et al (1977) and Nwuga (1982) noted that parity and age were associated with severer back pain in pregnancy.

This increased mobility is mediated hormonally. In 1926 Hisaw described a hormone which caused separation of the pubic symphysis in rodents, and showed that serum from pregnant guinea pigs caused relaxation of the pelvic ligaments when injected into virgin guinea pigs. The same team found the corpus luteum to be the source of the 'relaxation-causing factor' and named it Relaxin. The substance was found in humans and Weiss et al (1976) confirmed that it was produced by the corpus luteum. A report by Zarrow and McClintoch (1966) of relaxin being produced by the human decidua was confirmed recently (Bigazzi 1981, Bryant-Greenwood and Greenwood 1981, Larkin 1981). Relaxin receptor sites have been identified, and it seems that such sites must first be primed by oestrogen. At one time it was suggested that relaxin was target specific for the symphysis pubis, but from more recent animal work it seems probable that relaxin plays a role in the remarkable ability of the uterus to distend and in the formation of the collagenous framework for this. It inhibits contraction of smooth muscle and may play a part in cervical ripening. If this is so, withdrawal after delivery would assist involution. From animal studies it appears that the joint laxity is the result of the gradual breakdown of collagen in the target tissue and its replacement with a remodelled modified form with greater distensibility and pliability. The collagen synthesis is greater than collagen degradation, and there is an increased water content and so an increased volume.

Thus far, back pain in pregnancy has been approached from the medical model: that pain is organic, a bodily sensation, a biological signal of a threat to the structural or functional integrity of the person. Before leaving the causes of back pain in pregnancy it is worth considering it from the psychological aspect. Szasz (1957, 1968) describes two further levels of pain in addition to the biological one, the expression of pain as a fundamental way of asking for help, and the use of the word 'pain' in communication with many possible meanings and usages. The behaviourist school (Fordyce et al 1973) sees 'pain behaviours' — moaning, crying, stopping activity, clutching at a painful part — being used to communicate pain and usually resulting in sympathy and attention. Thus the behaviours themselves can become rewarding and inherently satisfying. A complaint of back pain could result in an anxious, fearful pregnant woman spending more time under the health care umbrella and being seen more frequently by a variety of professionals with resulting reassurance.

Some have tried to show that back pain is suffered by a certain personality group with an inference of inferiority. There is conflicting evidence as to which comes first, depression or back pain. Mantle et al (1981) found no evidence that depression preceded back pain in pregnant women. However, a pregnant woman may well experience additional stress, for example fear of labour, problems with employment, finance, housing or relationships. She is frightened to take pain killers, and a new unfamiliar pain heightens the universal anxiety about the welfare of the fetus, 'Is the baby alright?' In the author's experience, malingering is not a problem in this group of patients but the possibility must not be ignored.

Pain, whatever its cause, is itself a source of stress and is associated with irritability and anxiety (Moon 1981a); this in turn may cause severe changes in the sufferer's family and social relation-ships. For example, being unable to continue in work as long as planned may cause financial difficulties, and being unable to lift or care for other children may result in stress not only for the patient but for members of the family and friends. Stress is shown in body posture (Mitchell 1977): the body tends to adopt the instinctive 'fight or flight' pose. These positions, if held for any length of time or adopted habitually, will cause local and general fatigue. So a vicious circle is produced of pain, tension, fatigue, pain etc. Thus the reader has been taken a full circle back to fatigue as a possible cause of backache in pregnancy.

PREVENTION OF BACK PAIN IN PREGNANCY

Ideally, a woman should be as physically fit as possible before conception. However, the author has known of several women who, appreciating the need to improve their fitness, have chosen unwise types of training or placed themselves in untrained or inappropriately trained hands with disastrous results as far as their backs were concerned. Well Women's Clinics would do well to provide a suitable service. A physiotherapist — particularly an obstetric physiotherapist — is best equipped to individually assess the physical needs and prescribe and supervise appropriate regular exercise. If a woman has back problems before she becomes preg-nant it is important that all efforts are made to contain these prior to a pregnancy. But it must be emphasised that no inevitable correlation has been shown between back pain before pregnancy and back pain during a pregnancy. Much unnecessary suffering would be avoided if women had a basic understanding of simple biomechanics in relation to the spine and its usage. Instruction and advice in prophylactic back care should occur as part of primary and secondary education, be adapted to the work place, then be further reinforced early in pregnancy and related to childbearing and rearing. As little as two hours of instruction in early pregnancy has produced a significant reduction in the amount and severity of backache experienced in pregnancy (Mantle 1981). Such a prophy-lactic programme can be integrated into a comprehensive parent-craft preparation class system, but it is important that the groups are small enough to enable an informal, highly personalised service to be tailored to each individual's lifestyle and ergonomic problems.

The programme should commence with the opportunity to handle the bones of the spine and pelvis, and enable the client to begin to understand how movements occur and the forces associated with bending, twisting and lifting. Some appreciation of what is known of the causes of back pain in the non-pregnant and pregnant state is helpful. A convenient teaching vehicle is to take an average day from waking in the morning, through all the possible activities of the day, and back to bed for the night. Above all, comfort in bed, rest and sleep are important to a pregnant woman. Her increasing weight may cause even good quality beds to sag. Layers of blanket, towelling or newspaper under the mattress can prevent this. The knees crooked over a pillow will be more comfortable when supine lying. Most pregnant women increase their hip width with a pad of fat on the lateral aspect of the thighs. In side-lying, the normal sleeping position for most people, this greater width requires more rotation of the pelvis on the trunk in order to rest the upper leg on the bed. This increased rotation may cause pain and even strain lax sacro-iliac joints. The solution is to rest the top thigh on a pillow on the bed. When turning over in bed the knees should be flexed and held together to avoid sacro-iliac strain. In cases of restlessness or sleeplessness of either client or partner it may be appropriate to advise separate beds.

Pregnant women, particularly in the first and third trimester, experience frequency of micturition. This requires that they get in and out of bed more often at night, which is made more difficult by their increasing weight. The least stressful way to do this is to turn on to the side with knees flexed, drop the lower legs over the side of the bed and sit up sideways. This avoids the struggle to sit up forwards with repetitive jarring of the lumbar spine. The process should be reversed to get into bed. Dressing, washing hair, preparing meals, making beds and ironing provide a host of illustrative ergonomic problem areas and may be used to encourage clients to talk about their own circumstances and working environments. Working surface heights, avoiding twisting movements and standing with one foot in front of the other, are key teaching points.

A useful group activity can be conducted with 8 or 10 different chairs, ranging from easy to upright. The importance of a chair fitting the occupier and suiting the activity to be carried out is quickly appreciated, as is the means of making a chair more appropriate to the individual. Firm support in the lumbar region is an important factor in preventing and relieving back pain in pregnancy (Mantle 1977, 1981). The concept of good posture in standing, walking and sitting should be discussed, together with the possible progressive adverse effects of pregnancy and increasing lordosis. The simplest device is to encourage women to stand, walk and sit TALL. Understanding the role of the pelvis in posture is invaluable, and pelvic tilting should be taught in several positions, e.g. crook lying, sitting and walk-standing. Women are quick to grasp how the effects of fatigue and fitness, anxiety and contentment are mirrored in posture.

However, it is hard for a woman to appreciate early in her first pregnancy how it may alter her ability to lift and bend. Unless the habit of bending the hips and knees to stoop is formed by the end of the first trimester, it becomes progressively more difficult to establish, simply because the quadriceps muscles are not strong enough to raise the increasingly heavy body from the squat position. Heavy lifting should be avoided or shared. Carrying loads should be reduced to a minimum, and divided into two equal portions. Too long or too much of any activity or position can precipitate back pain. Women are encouraged to analyse retrospectively any back pain experienced with a view to avoiding pain-producing activities or ceasing such activity before pain begins.

It is helpful to discuss back care in relation to baby and child care. This prevents inappropriate purchases of baby equipment and encourages women to use the newly learned principles to their long-term benefit. In succeeding classes, other teaching methods may be used to give variety, for example slides or videos of good and poor positions or right and wrong methods of lifting. Active physical participation, practice and demonstration by group members is an important means of consolidating concepts and gives the opportunity for correction. Throughout, the obstetric physiotherapist is encouraging each woman to listen to her own body and so develop body awareness of comfort and well-being versus strain and fatigue. An additional means of achieving this is by training in neuromuscular control (relaxation) which should be included in all Parentcraft Programmes.

MANAGEMENT OF THE PATIENT WITH BACK PAIN IN PREGNANCY

Such management will be undertaken in close liaison with the rest of the obstetric team, and a full appraisal of the obstetric, as well as other, notes is essential.

The physiotherapist's care of a pregnant patient with back pain should, wherever possible, commence with a careful and thorough assessment. Occasionally, where pain is acute and/or there are contra-indicating signs, this must be delayed and a preliminary period of total or partial bed rest instituted. While it should never be assumed that the back pain is due to the pregnancy, the fact that the back pain sufferer is pregnant is of particular relevance in the assessment and treatment.

ASSESSMENT OF THE PATIENT

This will follow the classic pattern familiar to physiotherapists of assessment of a patient with back pain, but must be adapted to the pregnancy. The following comments illustrate this.

1. Subjective examination

a. Details of present pain

In addition to their back pain many pregnant women complain of abdominal 'stitch' pain and of pain around the costo-chondral margin, anteriorly, in the third trimester. Both are commonly attributed to pressure associated with the enlarging uterus and the lie of the fetus. When questioning patients, it must be appreciated that their chief concern will be the welfare of the fetus, not themselves.

b. Details of any other symptoms or signs

Here a thorough knowledge of the changes and course of normal pregnancy, and of possible complications, is imperative. For example, the pregnant body normally retains more fluid, and women in the third trimester frequently experience oedema of ankles and hands which is worse in the evenings and in hot weather, and is exacerbated by prolonged standing or walking. In the hands this can lead to a 'carpal tunnel' like syndrome with pins and needles. However, the obstetric physiotherapist must be fully aware of the possible serious implications of oedema and its relation to pre-eclamptic toxaemia.

c. Mandatory questions concerning the 'saddle area' and changes in micturition habits

The experienced obstetric physiotherapist will be able to distinguish between significant symptoms and the frequency, urgency and stress incontinence commonly experienced at various stages of pregnancy, also the considerable discomforts and changes in sensation of the perineum directly related to the pregnancy and caused by piles, venous thrombosis of the vulva or the weight of the fetus for example.

d. Onset and history of the episode

The stage of the pregnancy is highly relevant in that hormonal changes commence early and important enlargement and increase in weight comes later. Severe backache can occur in the final days of a pregnancy and can be the herald of labour.

e. General physical health, occupation and lifestyle

The total daily physical and mental load on the patient must be assessed.

f. History of previous episodes and any treatment received

There is no inevitability of pre-pregnancy episodes resulting in similar problems in a pregnancy, but an episode in a previous pregnancy is relevant (Calguneri 1982).

2. Planning the objective examination

Sensitivity and ingenuity are required in choosing positions of stability and comfort for the patient. It must be appreciated that changes in joint mobility may or may not be attributable to the pregnancy.

3. Objective examination

In the later stages of pregnancy the distended abdomen demands postural adaptations, and the lie of the fetus at a particular point in time can produce asymmetry of waist contours and even of shoulder levels. The 'strut effect' of the abdominal uterus limits all spinal movements. The heavily pregnant woman is less stable, and it may be helpful if, while being examined in standing, the patient faces a firm plinth on which she can lean for balance. A pregnant patient may become faint if kept in supine-lying for any length of time in later pregnancy, possibly due to pressure of the gravid uterus on the inferior vena cava; therefore this section of the examination should be conducted as speedily as possible. Should the patient feel unwell, the symptoms will disappear immediately if she turns on her side. The judicious use of pillows may allow prone-lying to be used for the final part of the examination, or alternatively side-lying may be preferred with a firm pillow at the waist.

4. Recording

In a clinical specialty area so prone to litigation it is prudent to be meticulous in record keeping.

5. Decisions regarding treatment

The patient should be included in the decision-making process in order that due weight may be given to the problems as perceived by the patient. The obstetrician should also be consulted in order that no obstetric considerations be omitted.

TREATMENT OF BACK PAIN IN PREGNANCY

The following modalities may be considered by the obstetric physiotherapist in the treatment of back pain in pregnancy:
1. Rest
2. Support
3. Postural and back care training and advice, body awareness and neuromuscular control
4. Manipulation
5. Traction
6. TENS
7. Heat
8. Massage
9. Exercise.

It has been shown that the addition of a passive modality to an active one produces better results and that symptomatic improvement increases with the number of treatment modalities used in combination (Coxhead et al 1981). Research into low back pain seems to indicate that manipulation, where possible, should be one of the modalities employed (Farrel and Twomey 1982, Edwards 1969), that back care training should be included (Bergqvist-Ullman and Larsson 1977) and that patients respond best where treatment is instituted early (Sims-Williams 1978). It must be remembered constantly that the placebo effect of any treatment, particularly where applied by a pleasant, efficient, professional therapist, is very powerful and can be expected to produce pain relief in up to 35% of cases.

There are some particular constraints on the treatment of the pregnant woman. Short wave diathermy to the trunk is contra-indicated, and it is generally agreed that interferential therapy should not be used. There has been reluctance on the part of some physiotherapists to use traction and manipulation, but in responsible hands they should be considered and could be an important component of treatment.

1. Rest

For acute debilitating back pain, bed rest for two or three days will almost always produce favourable results. Patients value some explanation for their pain, together with precise instructions as to how complete their resting should be. The obstetric psysiotherapist has an important role in helping the patient to find comfortable resting positions. In early pregnancy supported crook-lying can be used for moderated periods, but should be recommended only with extreme caution later in pregnancy because of the weight of the uterus which may compress main blood vessels. This can result in the patient losing consciousness, and there is a possibility of placental blood flow being impeded. Side-lying with a pillow between the knees or modified side-lying, quarter turned to prone, with the top leg and abdomen supported on pillows, are popular positions. The patient should be taught to turn over with knees crooked and pressed together, and how to get in and out of bed as previously described. Good sitting positions, diet, bowel movements and all other wise back care should be discussed.

It is important to establish that the patient is able to take the needed respite from her other responsibilities. It is sometimes necessary to take women into hospital to ensure they can rest or as a means of impressing on partners, families or employers that rest is really required. Rising unemployment has led to more women continuing in employment throughout their pregnancy, perhaps as the sole breadwinner of a partnership. Some employers are using market forces to exploit pregnant employees, even to the extent of refusing the legitimate entitlement of time off for clinic appointments. For rest to be effective all reasonable steps must be taken to avoid anxiety, guilt or frustration.

Back pain can occur in any individual if the work load or environment is sufficiently adverse. Some occupations are less suited to the pregnant woman than others. Sitting and standing for long periods and heavy manual work may predispose to backache. It may be entirely justified at times to insist on a woman ceasing employment or reducing activity in some way. Back pain can simply be the pregnant body indicating that it is being asked to do too much, and spectacular results can be achieved by reducing the stress level.

2. Support

It is accepted that there is no way of satisfactorily stabilising a hypermobile sacro-iliac joint or symphysis pubis short of sclerosis. The torsional strains of normal weight-bearing are too great. However, obstetric physiotherapists in several different parts of the world have found — apparently relatively independently — that a firm encircling pelvic support can bring relief without detriment to the fetus. In the United Kingdom Setons have produced the Fembrace to a physiotherapist's design. It is a length of sturdy elasticised material about 100 cm by 25 cm with Velcro ends, and is made in four sizes. It is applied in lying and taken across the sacro-iliac joints, passes down and forward to cross over, and fastens below the 'bulge'.

South African obstetric physiotherapists have developed a much narrower belt about 8 cm wide, made of soft leather, bound over and round a length of thick felt, laid on a length of buckram. Patients are encouraged to put it round the pelvis and fasten it tightly at whatever level and angle gives maximum pain relief. In Australia obstetric physiotherapists have adopted the Japanese maternity lumbo-sacral support, which women can make for themselves from 2 metres of fine cotton poplin fabric. The fabric is cut in half longitudinally and the two lengths are sewn together to produce a 4 metre length. This is folded in half longitudinally, the raw edges are sewn together and half an 8 inch elastic bandage is stitched to one end. The binder thus produced is wound firmly round the pelvis ending with the elastic portion and fastened with pins.

Conventional lumbo-sacral support belts can be worn in early pregnancy and maternity models can be individually tailored with an elastic front panel. Occasionally patients have benefited from the application of several layers of wide Tubigrip, but it is unlikely that it can offer any really effective support.

3. Postural and backcare training and advice, body awareness and neuromuscular control.

Broadly the instruction and advice will follow the prophylactic approach detailed earlier in this chapter. It will, of course, be precisely adapted to the history, symptoms and circumstances of the individual. Certain activities may have to be totally or temporarily vetoed, or made possible by means of a device, e.g. changing the height of a working surface, or taking a cushion to work to place in the small of the back when sitting. Other problems can be circumvented, e.g. rearranging kitchen cupboard contents to avoid repetitive stooping for the most commonly used items.

As the woman becomes more familiar with and sensitive to the feeling of her own body (body awareness) she will be able to detect, interpret, control and avoid harmful stresses, strains and fatigue. Where postural habits and body usage have to be changed the new positions and ways of doing things feel strange at first and take time to imprint, but the benefit is quickly evident. It is always valuable to teach back pain sufferers neuromuscular control (relaxation) to combat fatigue, as a means of training body awareness and as an actual 'at the time' stress coping mechanism. The Mitchell Method of Physiological Relaxation is favoured by many obstetric physiotherapists for this purpose. It is clearly documented in *Simple Relaxation* by Laura Mitchell published by John Murray.

4. Manipulation

Manual mobilisations and manipulations have been used successfully on pregnant patients with backache (Fraser 1976, Golightly 1982, Thomson 1986). The philosophies of these modalities emphasise the need for meticulous assessment and reassessment after every technique, and a competent physiotherapist will be able to interpret her findings in the light of the pregnancy. Backache in pregnancy may occur at any level, but is most prevalent in the lower lumbar and buttock region, occasionally with leg pain. All physiotherapists will have their preferences as to which techniques they find most satisfactory, but all must be guided by their findings. The most commonly used mobilisation technique for the lumbar spine in pregnancy is Grade 1 and 2 rotation. The side-lying starting position with the lumbar spine in the neutral position is ideal for transverse vertebral pressures which will ease facet joints, made irritable by increased degrees of lordosis. Postero-anterior central vertebral pressure may be useful up to the third and fourth month. Longitudinal movement to one or both legs may be effective at any stage. If the pain is thought to be associated with a forward torsion of a sacro-iliac joint, the ilium can be gently oscillated backwards on the sacrum by pressure applied to the ischial tuberosity and the anterior aspect of the ilium on the affected side with the patient in lying and the affected leg flexed at hip and knee. This can also be carried out as a manipulative thrust.

Where the signs and symptoms indicate a forward torsion of one ilium on the sacrum, Golightly and Fraser report successes with a manipulative technique devised by Cyriax to gap the appropriate joint, to enable it to return to a more normal approximation on release. The patient lies supine with the knee of the affected side flexed and the toes hooked under the straight knee. The therapist takes the flexed knee across the body while holding the shoulder of the affected side against the plinth. Thus tension is applied to the affected sacro-iliac joint and any slack is taken up. At the end of range the therapist applies a single gentle thrust. This manipulation should only be used when there is clear indication for it to attempt to correct malalignment. However, by the very nature of pregnancy the condition may recur. The manipulation should be performed as infrequently as possible or the soft tissues surrounding the joint may become overstretched. A Fembrace support may be applied following the manipulation.

Fraser also describes the simple, less severe manoeuvre which patients may perform for themselves once or twice a day to encourage the ilium to remain in a more normal position. It is described for the right sacro-iliac joint. The patient lies supine and grasps the right flexed knee at the level of the tibial tubercle with the right hand. The right hip is then rotated laterally sufficiently to allow the right calcaneum to be cupped in the left hand. With the trunk fully supported and the left leg relaxed and straight, the right knee is gently pulled toward the right shoulder and the right heel is eased toward the left groin. The pressure is then released. The movement is repeated once or twice.

5. Traction

Application of mechanical lumbar traction to a pregnant woman with back pain may seem, at first thought, unwise or even hazardous. In fact it can be achieved and has been used quite safely and comfortably, particularly in the first and second trimester. It should be considered for patients whose symptoms are referred into the legs, and where these have gradually appeared over a period of days or longer, in the absence of specific trauma. The patient may be treated in supine-lying or crook-lying. Having regard to the changes in the properties of connective tissue which may make distraction and movement of joints a little easier, small poundage only is used. As Grieve (1981), writing of traction in general terms, comments: 'Clinical experience teaches that relatively small poundage, sufficient to equal the natural opposition tendencies maintaining the integrity of resting joints, is often enough to relieve pain and limitation'.

6. TENS

Transcutaneous electrical nerve stimulation (TENS) involves the transmission of electrical energy across the surface of the skin and has its effect via the nervous system. Since the early 1970s it has been increasingly used all over the world to control pain of a variety of types and has been used successfully in the relief of pain in labour without harm to the fetus or the newborn (Augustinsson 1977, Bundsen and Ericson 1982). Though quite commonly used to relieve back pain in the non-pregnant, there are few recorded instances of its use for the purpose in pregnancy. However, Mannheimer (1985) reported two cases where it was used successfully and apparently safely, and the author's experience concurs with this.

TENS should only be used as a symptomatic means of pain control, as an adjunct of a carefully considered treatment programme. In pregnancy, particular caution is required with a modality capable of modifying the pregnant body's response to pain for some hours. However, for the properly selected case it may well be preferable to medication. The conventional stimulation mode i.e. high pulse rate (50–100 Hz), narrow pulse width (30–75 μs) and low amplitude (10–30 mA), is used. The patient is instructed in the use of a suitable machine and in the appropriate placing of the electrodes. A decrease in pain perception, thought to occur as a result of 'gating' of the painful stimuli at the dorsal horn of the spinal cord, is apparent quite quickly and commonly remains for about three hours. The patient is encouraged to experiment at home in the duration and frequency of application which gives the maximum pain relief. However, she must be fully cogniscent of all aspects of wise back care, be receiving other modalities of treatment if appropriate and have her condition regularly reviewed. She should appreciate that diminution of pain is *not* necessarily an indication that the condition is cured, nor that full normal activity may be resumed.

7. Heat

Heat may be applied for modest periods to the painful area of the back by means of an electric pad, hot water bottle or an infra red lamp quite safely, providing the skin sensation over the area is normal. The warmth is soothing and may have a beneficial influence on tissue fluid exchange in muscle and connective tissue. It also affects arterial, venous and lymphatic flow, and may relieve muscle spasm. There is no evidence that heat applied in this local superficial manner adversely affects the fetus. However, short wave diathermy is generally thought to be contra-indicated, even when applied superficially by means of a coil. Taking frequent hot baths to soothe backache may be contra-indicated in late pregnancy, especially where there is any predisposition to premature labour. A hot bath is a recognised means of encouraging the onset of labour and also accelerating its progress.

8. Massage

Massage is a neglected and under-used modality which, in practised hands, has considerable benefit for a painful back, with no adverse side-effects. Slow soothing stroking, effleurage and kneading, performed with the patient supported with pillows in side-lying or three quarter turned to prone-lying, combine to encourage relaxation — both general and local, relieve pain and muscle spasm and assist the circulation. Painful tissue, which has become stiff and even shortened, can be mobilised and stretched. Manipulation of soft tissue, as in kneading, is thought to stimulate the body to produce its own endorphins. It communicates care and concern, and enables the patient to experience positive pleasant stimuli from an area of the body from which she may have become alienated.

9. Exercise

Rest is usually the best therapy for the acute back but, once the symptoms subside, gradual mobilisation may be commenced. Gentle pelvic tilting in crook-lying is one of the earliest and most universally beneficial movements, and can relieve stiffness and spasm. It may be appropriate to attempt to strengthen weak muscle groups, particularly to enable good posture to be maintained. Occasionally, easy spinal exercises, commenced in non weight-bearing positions, are needed simply to assist the patient to regain confidence in her spine. But it must be remembered that the pregnant woman's body is increasingly under stress because of her continuing weight gain, thus there is a built-in progressive resistance to exercise. A judicious balance between rest and a variety of different positions and activities appears to be one of the secrets of success.

Warm water is a most appropriate and efficacious medium for the pregnant woman following an episode of back pain, and swimming, if pleasurable to the woman and agreeable to the obstetrician, may well constitute the perfect progression of exercise. The buoyancy of the water temporarily relieves the beleaguered joints. Indeed swimming pools are increasingly popular venues for antenatal classes (see Ch. 7).

THE FUTURE

The future management and prevention of this wretched condition, which so alters the quality of life, is inextricably bound up with developments in unravelling back pain as a whole. Backache in pregnancy constitutes just one facet, albeit an important one, of the total life-back-pain picture. For any individual it seems likely that a variety of factors and events are associated and accumulate to produce back pain. It has been the lot of many patients to suffer unbearable episodes of pain, yet have no clinically demonstratable abnormality to confirm and substantiate their complaint. Recent exciting developments in techniques which are able to image soft tissues have already exposed the explanation for the fortunate few. It is to be hoped that it will be possible to extend and reduce the cost of this valuable assistance, for it is helpful to both the carer and the patient to understand what is hurting and why. Therapy will then be more precise, and in the longer term so will research and prophylaxis. There is hope too in recent moves, such as the formation of the International Back Pain Society, to encourage collaboration between orthopaedic and neuro surgeons, specialists in rheumatology and rehabilitation, biochemists, biomechanical engineers, physiotherapists, psychologists, osteopaths, basic scientists and others in the pain field..

The endocrinologists may have a particular contribution to make to the alleviation of backache in pregnancy by researching further the hormones in relation to joint laxity, and their optimum levels. It may be that some pregnant women produce excess amounts of these, and this might prove to be controllable. If such control were possible, it would also benefit those who have sacro-iliac joint hypermobility before a pregnancy and for whom even the normal increase is a problem.

Until there is better understanding of the factors associated with back pain causation, back health must be vigorously pursued with logic and common sense, utilising all that is known of the properties and reactions of the body tissues, and of biomechanics. Their present training gives physiotherapists a comprehensive and appropriate core of knowledge and skill to enable them to be effective in back pain prevention, assessment and in therapy by physical means. In prophylaxis their potential is largely untapped. The health of a pregnant woman's back will be substantially dependent on the fundamental quality of the spinal structure and the mechanical 'fit' of the moving parts, which are factors largely determined before birth. But back health is also affected by general health, body usage, type of work, by injuries experienced and by the extra special strains of pregnancy and parturition. Physiotherapists, trained, as they all are, in teaching and the presentation of practical material are uniquely fitted to contribute to many aspects of health education, for example the promotion of back health in schools, colleges, Well Women's Clinics, fitness centres and antenatal classes. They also have a role in the design of buildings, furniture and other equipment, as well as in the assessment and improvement of working environments.

Finally, it is not hard to envisage that just as smoking is now condemned in the interest of chest health, so other aspects of the 20th century lifestyle may have to be modified in the interest of back health. Could it be that it is unreasonable for a person to sit at a keyboard for more than five hours a day? Should pregnant women be encouraged to stop work earlier than 28 weeks of pregnancy? Would it help for the UK to follow the French example of having a legal limit for loads carried by both female and male employees? The Back Pain Association is already appraising the care of children's backs throughout school life. Much careful evaluation is possible and required urgently to try to prevent the present huge quantity of back pain misery generally, and obstetric back pain specifically.

REFERENCES

Abramson D, Roberts S M, Wilson P D 1934 Relaxation of the pelvic joints in pregnancy. Surgery, Gynecology and Obstetrics 58:595

Augustinsson L E, Bohlin P, Bundsen P 1977 Pain relief during delivery by transcutaneous electrical nerve stimulation. Pain 4:59

Bergqvist-Ullman M, Larsson U 1977 Acute low back pain in industry. Acta Orthopaedica Scandinavica Supplement 170

Bigazzi M 1981 Relaxin. Proceedings of the First International Conference 1980 Greenwood F C et al (ed)

Bryant Greenwood G D, Greenwood F C 1981 Relaxin. Proceedings of First International Conference 1980 Greenwood F C et al (ed)

Bundsen P, Ericson K 1982a Pain relief in labour by transcutaneous electrical nerve stimulation: Safety aspects. Acta Obstetrica Gynaecologica Scandinvica 61:1

Bundsen P, Ericson K, Petersen L E, Thiringer C 1982b Pain relief in labour by transcutaneous electrical nerve stimulation: Testing of a modified stimulation technique and evaluation of the neurological and biochemical condition of the newborn infant. Acta Obstetrica Gynaecologica Scandinvica 61:129

Calguneri C, Bird H, Wright V 1982 Changes in joint laxity occurring during pregnancy. Annals of the Rheumatic Diseases 41:126

Coxhead C E, Inskipp H, Mead T W North W R S, Troup J D G 1981 Multicentre trial of physiotherapy in the management of sciatic symptoms. The Lancet, May 16, 1065

DonTigny R L 1985 Function and pathomechanics of the sacro-iliac joint. Physical Therapy 65(1):35

Edwards B C 1969 Low back pain resulting from lumbar spine conditions: a comparison of treatment results. Australian Journal of Physiotherapy 15:104

Farrell J P, Twomey L T 1982 Acute low back pain. Australian Medical Journal. Feb. 20:160

Fordyce W E, Fowler R S, Lehmann J F, De Lateur B J, Sand P L, Trieschmann R B 1973 Operant conditioning in the treatment of chronic pain. Archives of Physical Medicine and Rehabilitation 54:399

Fraser D 1976 Post partum backache; a preventable condition? Canadian Family Physician. 22:1434

Golightly R 1982 Pelvic arthropathy in pregnancy and the puerperium, Physiotherapy 68 (7):216

Grieve E 1980 The biomechanical characterisation of sacro-iliac joint motion. M Sc thesis, University of Strathclyde

Grieve G P 1981 Common vertebral joint problems. Churchill Livingstone, Edinburgh, p 398

Hagan R 1974 Pelvic girdle relaxation from an orthopaedic point of view. Acta Orthopaedica Scandinavica 45:550

Hisaw F L 1926 Proceedings of the Society for Experimental Biology and Medicine 23:661

Larkin L 1981 Relaxin. Proceedings of First International Conference 1980 Greenwood F C (ed)

Lewit K, Knobloch V, Faktorova Z 1970 Vertebral disorders and obstetric pain. Manuelle Medizin 4:79

Lewit K, Wolff H D 1970 Conference on the pelvis. Manuelle Medizin 6:150

Mannheimer J S 1985 TENS — uses and effectiveness. In: Hoskins Michel T (ed) Pain. International Perspectives in Physical Therapy. Churchill Livingstone, Edinburgh, p 77

Mantle M J, Greenwood R M, Currey H L F 1977 Backache in pregnancy. Rheumatology and Rehabilitation 16:95

Mantle M J, Holmes J, Currey H L F 1981 Backache in Pregnancy II: Prophylactic influence of backcare classes. Rheumatology and Rehabilitation 20:227

Meckel J F 1816 Handbuch der Menschlichen Anatomie, Vol 2. Halle and Berlin

Mitchell L 1977 Simple relaxation. John Murray, London

Moon M H 1981a Post-operative pain: EMG biofeedback measures and relaxation. Proceedings IXth International Congress of Physical Therapy, Sweden

Nwuga V C B 1982 Pregnancy and back pain among upper class Nigerian women. Australian Journal of Physiotherapy 28:4

Sashin D 1930 A critical analysis of the anatomy and pathological changes of the sacro-iliac joints. Journal of Bone and Joint Surgery 12:891

Sims-Williams H, Jayson M I V, Young S M S, Baddeley H, Collins E 1978 Controlled trial of mobilisation and manipulation for patients with low back pain in general practice. British Medical Journal 2:1338

Szasz T S, 1957 Pain and pleasure. Tavistock, London

Szasz T S 1968 The Psychology of persistent pain. Academic Press, New York

Thomson A 1986 Middlesex Hospital School of Physiotherapy, London. Personal communication

Weisl H 1955 The movements of the sacro-iliac joint. Acta Anatomica 23:80

Weiss G, O'Bryne E M, Steinetz P G 1979 Science. 194:148

Zarrow M X, McClintock J A 1966 Journal of Endocrinology 36:377

Aspects of body learning for the childbearing year

INTRODUCTION

Various controversies have surrounded the question of activity in pregnancy. Llewellyn-Jones has said of the pregnant woman: 'She should not alter her regimen of exercise just because she is pregnant.' Elizabeth Noble on the other hand has devoted a book to a programme of exercise for the antenatal and postnatal periods. As long ago as the 1930s Dr Fairbairn (see Introductory chapter) wrote: 'In view of the advantages of special physical training for athletic contests, it seems reasonable that some form of preparation might serve to fit the expectant mother for the task before her.'

In recent years, two trends have led to an increased interest and demand for physical training in the antenatal period. One is the enormous interest generally in fitness, the other is the Active Birth Movement. The latter has grown largely out of pressures from women who wish to participate more fully in their labours. In order for this participation to be effective, a woman needs to be physically fit and practised in the positions she may choose for delivery. This may involve squatting — a difficult posture for most Western women. She also needs to develop a sensitivity to her own body so that she is able to respond to the relevant messages. In this chapter it will be seen that body learning encompasses relaxation and breathing awareness as well as movement, in order to attain the desired result. It is important that physiotherapists, and particularly those who specialise in obstetrics, should undertake this training. The increased body weight, and especially the ligamentous laxity caused by hormone changes during pregnancy, create a vulnerability of which the untrained teacher may be unaware.

Although this chapter is primarily related to childbirth, much of the advice could have a wider application, for example in preconceptual clinics. In the following pages a general description of the various components of body learning is followed by a section devoted to practical instructions related to each. The chapter ends with a suggestion of how this learning can help the woman in labour and through the postnatal period. Throughout, the term student should be understood to refer to anyone, including the pregnant woman, who wishes to learn.

POSTURE AND POSITIONING

It has been said that, correctly performed, standing, sitting and walking give the right form of exercise for 16 hours a day; wrongly performed they constitute strain and stress. Correct resting in lying for the remaining 8 hours should be added to this. Bad posture and movement can have an adverse effect on the body, while correct usage results in a sense of well-being.

To be given definite rules to develop good posture when individual body structures vary anatomically is questionable and could result in over-emphasis and stiffness. However, guidelines (see page 97) could be described as a series of images to develop instinct and inner feel. The concept of posture applies to lying, standing, sitting and moving.

Lying is a helpful starting position for acquiring a sense of the correct alignment of the body. It is frequently taught by physiotherapists when treating post-operative patients as a preliminary to standing. Standing for long periods can be a problem as man is designed to *move*. However, strains can be minimised by applying certain principles of joint positioning and by developing postural sensitivity. Sitting presents problems often caused by the bad design of chairs. Fortunately, chair manufacturers are beginning to realise the advantages of using the advice of physiotherapists in this field. It is important for the chair to have a firm high back to support the spine and preserve its natural curves. Robin McKenzie, in his book *Treat Your Own Back*, recommends a supportive roll positioned to maintain the lumbar curve.

Posture in pregnancy is affected by increasing body weight resulting in an alteration in the centre of gravity, and ligamentous laxity caused by hormone changes. Backache can result, and prophylactic advice given as early as possible in pregnancy lays particular stress on posture and positioning (Ch. 5).

NEUROMUSCULAR CONTROL

Tension is the natural reaction of the body to dangerous and/or painful situations — the 'fight or flee' response — a necessary protective reflex. If it is converted into action — running away or fighting back — the tension is released naturally. Unfortunately in many situations, particularly in the frustrations of urban life, this conversion does not take place and the tension builds up to a condition of stress. Laura Mitchell in her book *Simple Relaxation* quotes the astounding expenditure on sedatives and tranquillizers in the United Kingdom for the year 1979 as £43 980 000. Today, the mushrooming of classes in yoga and transcendental meditation etc. indicates the demand for a more healthy solution to the problem.

Childbirth is potentially an event of great anxiety and in the 1930s the obstetrician Grantly Dick-Read recognised in the labouring woman a syndrome of fear causing tension causing increased pain. He sought to break this cycle by teaching antenatally relaxation and a programme of education in the events of child-birth. At an even earlier date, Minnie Randell was including relax-ation in her parentcraft classes at St Thomas' Hospital (see Introductory chapter). Throughout the various changes that have occurred since that time relaxation has remained an important component of antenatal preparation, and the Mitchell Method of Physiological Relaxation is the one most favoured by obstetric physiotherapists.

The aim of teaching relaxation is to achieve an altered physical response to pain through acquired skills. It is necessary to build up the student's confidence and convince her that if she is fit and relaxed she will more easily withstand the exigencies of labour and that ease and fear cannot exist together. 'All our natural bodily functions work better in a state of relaxation.' (Kitzinger 1984). Attitudes affect reactions; negative attitudes can result from the superstitions and mystiques surrounding childbirth. Anxiety and tension can become a habit which impairs respiration and body alignment; equally, once the skill has been acquired, relaxation can become a habit which can have benefits far beyond the childbirth situation.

BREATHING AWARENESS

Emotions affect respiration — equally respiration can affect the emotions. It can be of life-long benefit to develop an awareness of the rhythms and levels of breathing. An early study assessing the elaborate breathing patterns in the psychoprophylaxis method of labour training (see Introductory chapter), revealed that controlled breathing caused increased tension and stress. Recent work in Oxford further supports this view. 'It is likely that the mother's physiology knows best during labour, and that a better pattern of breathing that they could be taught, does not exist.' (Stradling 1983).

EXERCISE

Having achieved body awareness through training in posture, relaxation and breathing, the student can proceed to schemes of exercise or movement. The aims related to childbirth are:

1. To minimise the strains on the body caused by the changes in pregnancy and create a feeling of physical well-being.
2. To prepare for labour with special reference to positions for delivery.
3. To lay the foundation for postnatal recovery by developing an awareness of the muscles to be strengthened, particularly the abdominal and pelvic floor muscles.

Exercise for the abdominal muscles should be part of an antenatal programme to promote general physical fitness, but movements which overstretch the fibres must be avoided. The rectus abdominis is particularly vulnerable, with diastasis developing as the pregnancy progresses. This, if it persists to any marked degree postnatally, calls for special treatment by the physiotherapist. Slack abdominal muscles can contribute to the slumped posture of pregnancy and its consequent problems as described by Mantle (Ch. 5). Early posture training, with an explanation of the significance of the abdominal muscles, is probably the best way to preserve them and lay the foundation for postnatal recovery. An appeal to vanity can be very effective by using a full-length mirror to show the different sideways silhouette between the slack and held abdominal corset.

In Chapter 9, Shepherd describes the musculature of the pelvic floor, the problems which arise from weakness of this most important structure and how these are frequently associated with childbearing. The efficiency of the pelvic floor is diminished in pregnancy due to hormone changes and the increasing weight of the developing fetus. The postnatal condition and function of the muscles are affected by the continuing hormonal imbalance and the nature of the delivery. It has yet to be shown whether current second stage techniques (upright positions to increase the pelvic outlet and non-forced pushing) will have long-term beneficial effects on the pelvic floor, and these effects must also be considered when discussing the controversies surrounding the practice of episiotomy. It is vital for the pregnant woman to have an understanding of the function of the pelvic floor and to practise contractions regularly. This will give her an awareness of the muscles and an ability to relax them adequately during the second stage of labour and also promote a useful habit of exercise for the postnatal period. The importance of the condition of the pelvic floor related to the life-long health of a woman cannot be over-estimated. The physiotherapist must not miss the opportunity of imparting this essential ingredient of a health education programme.

PRACTICAL SECTION

The exercise schemes to follow are directed to the student, therefore the present tense is used. It is important to note that lying flat on the back may be an uncomfortable and ill-advised position for the pregnant woman, and therefore adaptations of some of the starting positions may be necessary. In the posture section the approach throughout should be dynamic — moving around each position before adopting the correct one — for example rocking the pelvis, rolling the head on the neck. In this way the spring and resilience of the joints will be appreciated. In the exercise section, mention of the number of times for each exercise has been purposely avoided. The build-up should be gradual and will vary with different individuals. Overtiring, particularly in pregnancy, must be avoided.

Posture

Posture in lying

The starting position is crook-lying with the feet flat on the floor or bed beneath the knees, a hip-width apart. The head is positioned on a 2-inch high support giving the correct alignment of the cervical spine.
1. Think about the knees directed towards the ceiling and the forehead reaching towards the ceiling — let go, do not hold.

2. Lower the back and feel gravity working on it — releasing the spine.
3. Feel the hammock effect of the body between the head and knees.
4. Carry the arms slowly out to the side, then bend the elbows and bring the hands to rest on the upper abdomen, keeping the elbows on the floor.
5. Feel the shoulders widening and supported by the floor and the chest expanding and relaxing.
6. Slowly straighten first one leg and then the other — moving on an out-breath and feeling the changed position.

To stand up

Bend both knees and roll onto the right side keeping the knees gripped together (this is important in pregnancy to protect the sacro-iliac joint) and push up into four-point kneeling. Move back into kneel-sitting. Keeping the spine and head in the alignment already established in lying, slowly stand and maintain good posture.

Posture in standing

Awareness of weight distribution in standing is through a triangle of the heel, base of great toe, base of little toe.
1. Feel the knees loose, mobile and off full-lock.
2. Feel the hips level.
3. Feel the pelvis free and mobile with no tension in the abdomen or lumbar region. The anterior superior iliac spines should be in the same plane as the pubic bone. (This should be so throughout the changes in pregnancy and constitutes a check of continuing correct posture.)
4. Visualise the spine as a spring — neither compressed nor over-stretched but released and open.
5. Extend the space between nipple and hip to give a correct positioning of the thorax.
6. Roll the shoulders easily and freely.
7. Hold the head as if the middle hairs were attached to the ceiling.
8. Now forget the body and take your head for a walk — feel the lightness and spring at each step and the alignment of head and spine.

Posture in sitting

The student should choose an appropriate chair as described on page 94.

1. Place the weight of the body centrally with the spine supported.
2. Keep the head aligned and poised.
3. Feel the thighs supported.
4. Position the legs angled slightly outwards freeing the hips.
5. Keep the feet flat on the floor directly beneath the knees.

Moving from sitting to standing

1. Keep the head in line with the trunk and lean forward from the base of the spine.
2. Do not hollow the back or crumple the neck — feel the shoulders at rest.
3. Imagine a thread through the top of the head and, maintaining the alignment of head and spine, feel the body being drawn forward and upward continuously until the buttocks leave the chair. Continue the movement to the standing position using the legs as the force.

Moving from standing to sitting

1. Imagine being drawn down by the base of the spine, keeping the head and spine in alignment.
2. Move slowly, allowing the knees to bend until the buttocks reach the chair.
3. Resume the correct sitting position, drawing up the head and trunk as described above.

Neuromuscular control

The following points will help the student who should refer to Laura Mitchell's *Simple Relaxation* for detailed instructions. The best starting position is supine-lying on a firm base with the head slightly raised. In pregnancy half-sitting may be more appropriate. Once the skill has been mastered it can be practised in various positions — see page 104 for relaxation postures for labour.

1. Practise with a sense of purpose, enjoyment and achievement.
2. Choose to practise and concentrate — if thoughts wander, emotional conflict blocks achievement.

3. Practise regularly — it takes time to re-programme the body's responses.
4. Feel how relaxation re-charges the batteries of the body, increasing energy levels.
5. Apply the technique to every-day situations — such as car-driving, typing. The Mitchell Method leads to an appreciation of the resting positions of all the joints in the body and the prevention of energy waste through tense postures.

Breathing awareness

The starting position is sitting (a) on a chair with correct support or (b) cross-legged on the floor.
1. Go through the relaxation already learnt, checking the ease position of each joint.
2. Follow the natural flow of air in and out of the body.
3. Focus attention at nostril level — feel the cold air entering and the warmer, moistened air leaving.
4. Take the attention to the back of the throat and follow the flow of air down to the bases of the lungs.
5. Feel how the waist and upper abdomen move out as the diaphragm descends on the in-breath and sink in as the air is expelled.
6. Notice the slight expansion sideways of the lower ribs as air is taken in and a caving-in as it is expelled.

Normal, natural breathing is a combination of these actions — the air reaching low into the lung bases. Conditions of anxiety and tension may disturb this rhythm and result in a shallower and quicker pattern of breathing.

Exercise

Exercises in lying (see page 97 for note re-lying in pregnancy)

1. Crook-lying — the legs hip-width apart, knees bent and feet flat on the floor. Tilt the pelvis, bringing the pubic bone nearer the ribs using the abdominal muscles and moving the lumbar spine into contact with the floor. Now reverse the movement, hollowing the back (pelvic rocking).
2. Crook-lying — raise the pelvis slowly so that the body approaches a straight line between the shoulders and knees. Lower slowly.

3. Crook-lying — draw the heels near to the buttocks and stretch the arms out sideways on the floor. Let the knees swing to the left, lowering them to the floor and keeping the shoulders in contact with the floor. Bring the knees back to the midline. Alternate from one side to the other in a continuous rhythmical movement.

4. Crook-lying — repeat Exercise 3, turning the head in the opposite direction to the movement of the knees — feel the gentle twist to the spine.

5. A somewhat unusual position — lying with legs up the wall. To assume it sit sideways next to the wall with the knees bent and feet flat on the floor. Swing round so that the legs go up the wall and the body is flat on the floor with the buttocks close to the wall. Have a small support under the head. Feel the legs extended and the knees loose and the lower back in contact with the floor.

   a. Move the feet up and down and then circle them at the ankles.
   b. Widen the legs apart as far as possible against the wall, easing into the position of stretch gently.
   c. With the legs hip-width apart, bend the knees keeping the feet flat on the wall, move the arms slowly above the head until they reach the floor. Relax into this position of stretch and hold it.
   d. Bring the soles of the feet together, lower the arms, and with the hands press gently on the knees pushing outwards. To move out of the position, bend the knees, roll over to one side, kneel and then stand.

Stretching postures in floor sitting

Sitting on the floor may be uncomfortable at first, but if practised a little and often these positions will gradually strengthen the back muscles and stretch tight tissues. A cushion under the pelvis may help to prevent a roll back onto the coccyx, or try sitting supported against a wall.

1. Sit cross-legged and change the front leg from time to time.
2. Sit in the tailor position with the soles of the feet together.
3. Sit with the legs out straight and wide apart.

In all the above positions keep the correct alignment of spine and head. It may help at first to place the hands on the floor behind the hips for support. Gradually increase the stretch on the inner thighs by allowing gravity to work on the knees in (1) and (2) and widening the legs apart in (3). Squatting should be practised regularly. At first it may be necessary to use a chair as support or to support the back against a wall. During pregnancy, squatting rather than bending the back for doing jobs low down or for lifting is particularly important (Ch. 5).

Exercises in kneeling

Kneel with the knees slightly apart, the back upright and head in alignment.
1. Stretch the arms to the ceiling with hands interlocked.
2. Place hands on the hips and rock the pelvis to and fro. Now change to a hip rolling movement in both directions.
3. Place the right foot flat on the floor in front of the right hip with the knee at a right-angle. Hold onto a support with the right hand. Sway the body forward over the right leg, bending the knee further and stretching the left leg while keeping the back straight. Change legs and repeat.

Exercises in prone-kneeling

Place the hands directly under the shoulders and the knees under the hips.
1. Arch the spine, rounding it towards the ceiling and bending the head towards the knees. Then lower the back raising the head (avoid hyperextending the lumbar spine in pregnancy). This can be combined with breathing as follows: breathe in and then breathe out as the back is arched, then in as the back is lowered. Do this rhythmically in time with natural breathing.
2. Move the pelvis, bringing the left hip towards the left shoulder and looking in the direction of the left hip. Repeat towards the other side.
3. Move forward placing the forearms on the floor. Rock the pelvis backwards and forwards.

Exercises in standing

Stand in corrected posture (see page 98), with knees shoulder-width apart.
1. Swing both arms forward and upwards rising on the toes, then lower arms and heels. This should be a rhythmical movement with arms and shoulders loose.

2. Feel the knees loose and off full lock and place hands on hips. Gently tilt the pelvis backwards and forwards like a belly dancer, then give a gentle hip roll in both directions.
3. Place hands on hips with thumbs behind, stretch the spine with head aligned and move forward from the hips keeping the back straight, then return to upright position.
4. As above, bend trunk sideways to the right, return to upright position and repeat to left.
5. As above, arch spine a little, pressing thumbs into back. Return to upright position.

Exercise for the pelvic floor

(May be practised in sitting or standing — always with a slight gap between the knees to prevent adductor action.)

Tighten the ring of muscle around the anus (as if stopping a bowel action) and tighten deep in the vagina (as if stopping the passage of urine). Combine the above and lift the whole tightened muscle drawing upwards, and hold it for four seconds. Relax slowly.

LABOUR

An essential ingredient of a preparation for childbirth programme is education in the events of pregnancy, labour and the puerperium. Ideally this should involve different members of the obstetric team and include both expectant parents. There should be ample time for discussion and an opportunity to see the labour unit. The couple will need to know which forms of artificial pain relief are available and the policy of the particular unit regarding such matters as positioning for delivery. The demands of women who wish to be involved in the management of their labour may present problems for the obstetrician and midwife whose priority has to be the safe delivery of a healthy baby. Realistic antenatal education with some stress on the unpredictability of labour and a caring team at the birth, can lead to a fulfilling experience for the mother, regardless of the nature of delivery.

First stage

Remaining upright and mobile in early labour may or may not

affect progress, but it certainly suits most women. In many units it is encouraged unless contra-indicated on medical grounds. The woman may wish to rest and relax during contractions assuming any of the following positions:

1. Standing leaning forward onto a table or against a wall or held in an embrace by her partner as she rests her head on his shoulder.
2. Sitting leaning forward onto her folded arms against a table or astride a chair resting on its back.
3. Kneeling, sitting on her heels and leaning forward with arms and head resting on a chair.

(All positions should be with legs apart and hips slightly flexed.) Her training in body awareness will guide her into the most comfortable position. Pelvic rocking or rolling may ease the discomfort of the contractions, also lower back massage by her partner. As the contractions become stronger it will be necessary to take positive action to prevent a build up of tension. This is done by applying the relaxation and calm breathing learnt antenatally. The support of the labour ward staff and the presence of the partner are important factors at this time.

Second stage

Changed attitudes towards positions for delivery are based on the work of J. G. B. Russell and others advocating a return to the natural primitive postures. Russell found an increase of 28% in the pelvic outlet between the supine and squatting position, as well as a mechanical advantage during the expulsive phase. Again, body learning and sensitivity will help the woman to adopt the most comfortable position, and prenatal exercise will help her to tolerate the position with the minimum strain. Forced pushing and breath-holding are probably best avoided as being exhausting and counterproductive. But the antenatal educator must be in constant communication with the labour ward staff so that all teaching is related to the delivery techniques of the midwives.

THE PUERPERIUM

A major benefit of the whole programme described in this chapter can be seen in the postnatal period. The priorities for the new mother are rest, sleep and exercise, graduated according to recovery and strength. However, there is a far bigger priority — the new baby. The mother has many new skills to learn to supply the baby's various needs (and if she intends to breast feed, time and effort are required especially for the first-time mother). She has to relate to the baby emotionally, which should be a joy but may present problems, and adjust to a completely changed lifestyle. In fact she is often considered to be the busiest client the physiotherapist meets, and it is vital that the approach to postnatal rehabilitation is completely realistic. She is unlikely to have the time and motivation to perform an adequate programme of formal exercise.

However, if the new mother has followed the suggested scheme of antenatal training, the habits formed will be invaluable to her during the early weeks following delivery. It is the role of the obstetric physiotherapist to encourage these habits, reminding the mother to integrate them into her busy day. Relaxation can help her to get the maximum benefit from any rest she can take as well as saving her energy by economy of muscle action. She will have learnt the correct resting and working postures and will adapt these to her new conditions. She will protect her back by arranging correct heights for working surfaces, for example nappy-changing, often best done in kneeling with the baby on the floor. She will adopt the most comfortable sitting position with back supported and shoulders in the resting position for feeding the baby. This will help mother and baby, for if the mother is tense the baby feels it and feeding is affected — especially breast feeding. The weakened muscles to be considered are those of the pelvic floor and abdomen. Ideally, the woman will have already developed the habit of contracting the pelvic floor regularly, and be aware of the vital importance of strengthening these muscles. Habits of correct posture (standing and walking tall) will be good for her back and start to strengthen the abdominal corset.

As the weeks pass the mother will become gradually accustomed to her new role and there will come a period when she has time to think of herself. Postnatal support groups in hospital or the community are invaluable and, where possible, should involve the obstetric physiotherapist. More advanced exercises can be taught, checks made to ascertain the strength and recovery of the pelvic floor, and any necessary advice given over problems such as backache. Incontinence and back problems in later life frequently relate back to the childbearing period. A comprehensive programme such as is described in this chapter should help to prevent such problems and result in body awareness and sensitivity leading to life-long benefits.

REFERENCES

Dick-Read G 1969 Childbirth without fear. Pan Books, London
Fairbairn J S 1934/35 Changes in thought in a half century of obstetrics. Transactions of the Edinburgh Obstetrical Society: 63–82
Kitzinger S 1984 The experience of childbirth, 5th edn. Penguin Books, London
Llewellyn-Jones D 1986 Fundamentals of obstetrics and gynaecology, 4th edn. Faber & Faber, London
McKenzie R 1980 Treat your own back. Spinal Publications, Waikanae, New Zealand
Mitchell L 1985 Simple relaxation. John Murray, London
Nobel E 1982 Essential exercises for the childbearing year, 2nd edn. Houghton Mifflin, Boston
Randell M 1945 Training for childbirth. J & A Churchill, London
Russell J G B 1982 The rationale of primitive delivery positions. British Journal of Obstetrics and Gynaecology 89: 712–715
Stradling J 1983 Respiratory physiology in labour. Journal of the Association of Chartered Physiotherapists in Obstetrics and Gynaecology 53: 5–7

Pregnancy and recovery: the aquatic approach

INTRODUCTION

It seems logical to want to remain in shape during pregnancy by
swimming and exercising in water. Indeed, it is a well-known fact
that swimming is the best all round exercise during pregnancy. It
is excellent for building up stamina, strength and suppleness whilst
the back is being relieved from strain. An additional advantage is
that pregnant women do not feel uneasy about their size and shape
once they are in the water so that they can swim without self-
consciousness.

Water has always inspired man: it was our natural environment
before we were born. The infinite power of waves smashing onto
rocks fascinates us, and everyone is familiar with the ultimate sense
of well-being of soaking in a nice hot bath. Swimming brings back
something of the holiday atmosphere. Water is a most playful
element that will never stop attracting and challenging us at the
same time.

These elements have been excellently made use of in France
where gynaecologists, midwives, swimming teachers and physiotherapists together worked out a schedule of exercises adapted to the
special needs of women before and after the birth of their baby.
This led to the establishment of the 'Association Nationale Natation et Maternité' (ANNM)*, an association involving all
professionals working in water with pregnant women.

ANNM

History

In France, childbirth preparation classes are given by midwives.
One midwife at the maternity hospital of Aulnay-Sous-Bois (Paris),
Mrs Estable, was often asked during her classes by pregnant

* ANNM 2Ibis, rue de la Marne. 93360 Neuilly Plaisance. France.

women whether they could continue swimming during their pregnancy. Mrs Estable, who herself had been swimming all through her pregnancies, formed the habit of accompanying the women and they very much enjoyed those weekly sessions. Since swimming lengths was tiring, the women rested in between, and gradually Mrs Estable started suggesting exercises to relax during those periods of rest and it became obvious that even bigger advantages could be derived from these sessions in the pool by creating a programme of adapted exercises.

In 1974, Mr Pommat, director of the pools in Versailles, was interested in this activity and set aside one hour a week for the exclusive use of the pool by pregnant women. With Mr Vallet, a physical education teacher and initiator of baby swimming in France, and Dr Bardiaux, gynaecologist in the hospital of Aulnay-Sous-Bois, they planned a fully adapted programme. In 1977 the ANNM was founded, linking doctors, midwives, physiotherapists, swimming instructors and parents-to-be. Since then the ANNM has been growing steadily. Today more than 70 centres are affiliated and more than 1000 people have been trained.

In the meantime, interest in the preparation in water has been developing fast in other countries. Over the last couple of years the courses of the ANNM have been taken by participants from Belgium, Monaco, Sweden, Switzerland, Italy, Guadeloupe and Canada. The ANNM is also corresponding with Japan, Australia and Singapore. The idea is to establish an international federation of perinatal hydrotherapy with headquarters in Brussels.* This federation will endeavour to encourage the exchange of ideas concerning the benefits for pregnant women between the different affiliated countries of the world.

Aims

The main purpose of the ANNM is to group different professionals who, because of their competence in their field, can add to the well-being of the future parents, using water as a medium. The proposed programme aims to keep the expectant mother in good shape and prepare her physically as well as psychologically for the birth and postnatal recovery. The ANNM ensures quality control of the sessions, and studies the data received from the different centres in order to obtain a better knowledge of the consequences

---

*Now established: I.F.P.H. Zevenbronnenweg 26, 1640 Sint-Genesius-Rode, Belgium

of swimming and exercising in water for the woman and the fetus. Another purpose is to create and form technical teams necessary to spread the method, and courses are organised twice yearly. These are followed mostly by midwives and swimming instructors, but also by physiotherapists and gynaecologists, and deal with different topics in the field of obstetrics and aquatics.

Once a year a follow-up is organised for those people already certificated by the ANNM. Different subjects can be proposed and new ideas and suggestions shared. People bring videotapes from their centres and talk about their difficulties. On these occasions people can also become more involved in the Association and propose themselves as candidates for different offices that need to be filled. They can also join one of the commissions dealing with such responsibilities as 'documentation', 'research', 'pedagogics'. . . etc.

Today the Association is flourishing, and a steady evolution with improved programmes is taking place.

BENEFITS OF THE METHOD

Cardiovascular

Body changes during pregnancy and delivery

From the 6th week of pregnancy the plasma volume increases to reach a mean of 3680 ml (compared with the non-pregnant 2566 ml). The red cell volume increases proportionately less, which can be a potential cause of physiological anaemia. However, this imbalance is normally compensated for by the raised haemoglobin concentration in pregnancy. The increased blood volume leads to a 30–40% augmentation of the cardiac output from about the 14th week with a raised heartbeat of up to 15 beats per minute. The increased abdominal volume pushes the diaphragm upwards, bringing the heart into a more horizontal position and creating typical changes in the electrocardiograph.

Physiologically, the arterial blood pressure decreases slightly during the second trimester of pregnancy. In the last trimester an increase is often observed, but blood pressure should not exceed 140 mmHg (systolic) and 90 mmHg (diastolic). A higher blood pressure may indicate toxaemia with the possible danger of pre-eclampsia. This should be treated immediately it occurs, the treatment depending on the severity. Rest and salt restriction may be advised or even an accelerated delivery. The increase in blood volume is accompanied by an increased dilatation of the veins of the lower abdomen downwards, and may cause varicose veins, haemorrhoids or swelling of the legs. During labour the heart rate increases with each contraction, and the cardiac output may increase by as much as 30%. During contractions the systolic pressure may rise, but should return to normal values in the period between contractions.

Influence of swimming

The entire cardiovascular system is influenced by muscle exercise such as swimming. Due to contact with water below the temperature of the skin, a narrowing of the blood vessels in the skin takes place in order to maintain body temperature, which further affects circulation. The increase in oxygen demand due to muscle activity is answered by an increase in blood flow by the heart. The exercise of swimming during pregnancy trains the heart for the challenge of pregnancy itself, and the stress of the delivery. The leg movements of swimming can be beneficial due to the alternation between contraction and relaxation of the muscles involved, which can be important for the venous return and thereby for prevention of varicosities. A slight drop in heart rate before and after swimming sessions for pregnant women has been described by Ponsar-Landré (1985).

Respiratory

Body changes during pregnancy and delivery

The thorax expands in an antero-posterior direction because the diaphragm goes up approximately 4 cm and abdominal respiration becomes more difficult. Congestion of the lung mucosa may appear, though rarely, making gas exchange more difficult. The vital capacity, which is the maximum amount of air inhaled after a forced exhalation, does not change significantly (Fig. 7.1). The tidal volume, the volume of gas inhaled and exhaled at one normal breathing cycle, rises slowly from the third month onwards to 40% of the normal value. There is an increase in the inspiratory capacity, and the functional residual capacity is reduced. Because the residual volume has a tendency to drop a decrease of total lung capacity may be found. Not only does the amount of air inhaled and exhaled with each breath increase, but also the rate of breathing: from about 15 to about 18 breaths per minute. With this

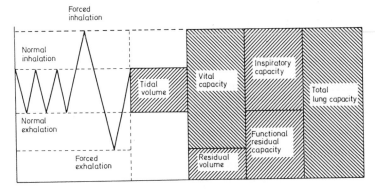

Fig. 7.1 The different volumes of ventilation.

slight physiological increase alveolar ventilation is improved.

During delivery, the respiratory cycle accelerates in direct proportion to the contraction in order to meet the vital need to excrete carbon dioxide. During expulsion, periods of apnea are alternated by periods of panting. Apnea may lead within a short while to hypoxia and hypercapnia.

During the process of delivery, metabolic acidosis may occur due to an over-production of lactic acid by the muscles, whose oxygen demand is temporarily increased and not answered appropriately by an increase in oxygen supply. In every instance of metabolic acidosis, the body answers with a respiratory effort to correct the acidosis, leading to compensatory respiratory alkalosis. The process of delivery is no exception to this physiological rule. Hyperventilation, being thus a physiological reaction to acidosis, is aggravated by the ample ventilatory movements during delivery. This leads to alkalosis, which has positive and negative effects. It diminishes consciousness a bit making the delivery less painful, but induces also a higher sensitivity to muscle spasms, which can lead to an increase in uterine tonus and cramps.

Panting has analgesic consequences; the uterus is not hampered by the contractions of the diaphragm. The problem is that the tidal volume is reduced, the amount of oxygen provided is insufficient and in the case of fetal distress this may be significant (Delecour 1985). The ideal situation would be to improve tidal volume while keeping the rhythm as steady as possible. To obtain maximum efficiency women have to be encouraged to breathe slowly and deeply during contractions. Panting can sometimes be of help, depending on the state of mind, for instance in case of panic in order to restore self-control, and to prevent occurrence of severe hyperventilation which induces respiratory alkalosis.

Influence of swimming

While swimming one learns to adopt a rhythmically synchronised breathing pattern. Whilst inhaling, the inspiratory muscles (intercostal and pectoral muscles) have to work against hydrostatic pressure, and because of the higher intra-abdominal pressure the lowering of the diaphragm requires more work. The exhalation has to be done in a very short time, and mostly against the resistance of the water. The simple fact of breathing with the body immersed thus tones up the respiratory muscles and diaphragm.

In competition swimming it has been found that the vital capacity improves. A vital capacity of 7 litres is no exception. This benefit has been taken advantage of in the re-education of patients with chronic respiratory insufficiency. Girardet (1978) studied 53 patients who followed the antenatal preparation classes in the pool and found a rise in vital capacity from 2.8 litres to 3.1 litres after six months.

Interviews with mothers who have followed this kind of preparation reveal the following concerning labour and birth (Ponsar-Landré 1985): the muscles are kept in good condition and the breathing is well co-ordinated. During labour the woman can fall back upon the known pattern of tranquil respiratory movements, improving the general relaxation. At the same time respiration can be associated with pelvic rocking as learned in the preparation, thus relieving painful tension in the small of the back, a defence mechanism against painful contractions (Baum-Sonnenschmidt 1982).

The relaxation exercises have also proved to be a great help. Some women consciously try to imagine they are relaxing in warm water in the pool and try to remember the different sensations accordingly. There is a better communication with the baby because of the regression to the previous fetal state. It has to be noted that in Belgium as well as in France this does not have to remain an imaginary experience: in certain hospitals mothers are allowed to relax and to deliver their baby in comfortably warm water (37°C). Other exercises have improved the suppleness of the adductors, allowing the woman to keep her knees apart without too much strain for a longer period of time if necessary. She has also learned consciously to release the pelvic floor muscles or to push the pelvic floor away and open up the vulva.

If necessary, periods of apnea can be sustained. The woman has learned to inhale after an exhalation in a very short period of time. The moments in between contractions can be fully used to relax and recover a regular breathing pattern. The efficient co-ordination of the respiratory rhythm, the effort of the expulsion and the releasing of the pelvic floor muscles, may shorten the period of expulsion considerably.

In Montpellier (Belaiche and Pistre 1984) and St Cloud (Renner 1985) studies have been done proving that exhaling against resistance, such as blowing up a balloon, is an effective means to relax the pelvic floor, leaving the straight abdominal muscles at rest, while the oblique and transverse abdominal muscles are fully called upon, wasting as little energy as possible.

Postural

Body changes during pregnancy

a. As the pregnancy proceeds, the abdomen expands, the centre of gravity is altered, and in order to maintain balance a series of compensatory body changes are developed.
b. The feet are placed more apart, thus broadening the supporting base, which results in a gait which is typical of the pregnant woman.
c. The weight of the abdomen causes the pubis to rotate downwards, resulting in an increased lumbar lordosis leading to an increase of all the natural curves of the spine.
d. The back muscles in the lumbar region are especially burdened and the ligaments weakened through the changed hormonal balance (Bardiaux 1984).
e. Hormonal action also affects the adipose tissues of thighs, buttocks and hips, causing retention of fluid.

Influence of swimming

The immersed body is virtually weightless, the back is unburdened and the warmth of the water adds to the relaxation of the tense muscles of the small of the back. The relief of back pain is often one of the major motives for the pregnant woman to come to the sessions. This relief can last for hours or days, and at times the problem disappears completely.

Psychological

During pregnancy and delivery

From day to day the future mother feels how her body expands and changes shape. She often feels enormous, unwieldy and unattractive, and may have to discontinue most of the sporting activities which added to her general feeling of well-being. More than ever during pregnancy she needs to feel comfortable and well in herself.

Influence of swimming

Swimming is the ideal sport for the pregnant woman. The warm water is an important aid to relaxation and the playful aspect of this form of preparation is also significant. The notion of body-weight is lost and this helps the woman to feel less self-conscious. She often feels more comfortable in the water than on an exercise carpet in a leotard. Another advantage of the sessions is that they seem to be an effective way of preventing insomnia, the women generally sleeping well the night after the session. During pregnancy bowel function is more difficult, adding to the physical and psychological sense of encumbrance. This bowel function is activated because of the exercises and the massage of the abdominal wall by the water.

CONTRA-INDICATIONS

A number of general contra-indications can be found:
a. Heart insufficiency.
b. Hypertension: immersion in water has been observed to influence the tension. Therefore each swimming session begins with the taking of blood pressure. If it is found to be too high, it is suggested the mother rests for a little while. If it remains high, she has to consult her doctor.
c. Respiratory insufficiency: certain cases of asthma, emphysema, chronic respiratory insufficiency, antecedents of spontaneous pneumothorax or pleurisy, tendency for lung fibrosis.
d. Tuberculosis.
e. Infections: sinusitis, bronchitis, ear or throat infections, vaginitis, urinary infections, skin disease or wounds.
f. Incontinence.
g. Epilepsy.
h. Diabetes.

Other contra-indications which are linked to the pregnant state are:
a. Toxaemia.
b. Danger of spontaneous abortion.
c. Cerclage for reason of dilated cervix. However, the systematic cerclage as a preventive measure, because of previous medical history, is not a contra-indication.
d. Antepartum bleeding.
e. Fetal hypotrophy and delay in intra-uterine growth.

It has to be noted that the risk of bacterial infection is minimal because of the strict sterilisation procedures used in public swimming pools.

MATERIAL ORGANISATION

The team of instructors

Most of the centres work with a team of at least a midwife and a swimming instructor, with the addition of a physiotherapist, gynaecologist, psychologist and paediatrician. Not all of them will be present at every session, but they will function as advisors. However, in France the presence of a midwife and a swimming instructor is strongly favoured (Ebersold-Estable 1984). The expectant mother will be met at the poolside by the midwife who takes her blood pressure. This is important because the blood pressure has been found to change when entering the water. It is also an extra opportunity to discover in time patients who are developing high blood pressure. Should the blood pressure be too high, the woman is asked to rest for a while on a bed in the first-aid room. If the blood pressure remains too high the woman will not be allowed to enter the water, and will be referred instead to her own doctor.

The midwife keeps records of details such as name, address, date of birth, expected date of delivery, weight, blood pressure, and in some centres the heartbeat, lung capacity and blood sugar. The intention has never been to stress the medical aspects of the activity, but to use this extra opportunity to monitor the pregnant women, to establish a personal link with them and to build in as much safety as possible. While these data are gathered the woman often reveals previously hidden feelings of fear or certain minor problems that can be easily solved with some advice. The woman relates to the midwife as a human being instead of a part of the sterile environment of the hospital. During the sessions the team observes the woman and notes any indication suggesting she is unwell and should come out of the water. In Belgium, where the activity has been spreading fast over the last few years, the sessions are mostly given by physiotherapists as it is they who do the antenatal preparation. Usually the blood pressure is not taken, because of lack of equipment.

After the women have seen the midwife, they are met in the water by a swimming instructor (or physiotherapist), and the session can start. Even if a physiotherapist is giving the sessions, it is wise to have a swimming instructor in the team. This is not only for reasons of safety and insurance but because they are the 'water specialists'. They tend to have a better didactical approach as they have more experience in teaching larger groups in this very specific environment. However, the courses offered by the ANNM also include theory and practice in the field of didactics, to teach midwives etc. how to relate to bigger groups in the water. Another advantage of having two people leading the session is that even more attention can be given to people with problems, for instance women who come for the first time and are not accustomed to the water.

The swimming pool

One of the concerns is the *temperature* of the water which should be high enough to allow relaxation and movements at a slow pace. The ideal temperature is from 30° to 32°C. If the water is too cold the stimulation threshold of the thermoreceptors in the skin is lowered and the motor neurons are stimulated, resulting in an increase of the muscle tone. If it is not possible to heat the pool up to 32°C, the movements have to be more vigorous and relaxing exercises have to be preceded by exercises concentrating on warming up. The *depth* of the pool is not very important, although it does determine the kind of exercises and materials used. Almost every exercise can be done in a depth of 1.50 m. In some centres only the small pool is heated sufficiently and the sessions take place in shallow water (from 20 to 80 cm) which considerably limits the choice of exercises. In Argenteuil* the women only use water in which they are out of their depth. Even women who cannot swim take part in these sessions as a network of ropes is stretched across the pool about 50 cm above the surface, which at any point the

*Desport, Centre Nautique. Argenteuil.

women can hold. Also, various floating materials in the form of boards, mats, balls etc. can be used. Ideally, the pool is used exclusively by the pregnant women as this adds to the tranquillity and peace of the session.

Frequency of the sessions

Lessons are mostly held once a week, but a few centres offer an additional session. Sometimes there is one hour provided each week, during which a woman can repeat activities from an earlier session by herself, and can relax in pleasant, warm water.

After the sessions

If possible, the women gather together after the sessions to chat with a cup of cocoa. This restores the blood-sugar level and at the same time they can share fears and problems and get to know each other better. Thus a valuable support system is created.

THE SESSIONS: PRACTICAL ORGANISATION

Exercise goals

The exercises proposed have four main goals:
a. Improvement of body awareness
b. Relaxation
c. Gentle shaping up
d. Breathing.

It is obvious that these particular aspects are not dealt with in an isolated manner, but various items are usually linked within one exercise. For example, the woman is in a prone position in the water, arms and legs relaxed. In this position she can contract and release the muscles around vagina and anus. This exercise improves her awareness of the pelvic floor muscles which prepares her for the second stage of labour. At the same time she can concentrate on complete relaxation of the rest of her body. Once she has mastered this she can proceed to co-ordinate it with her breathing — exhalation aiding the relaxation process (Fig. 7.2).

a. Body awareness

Most women learn to do the breast stroke when they are taught

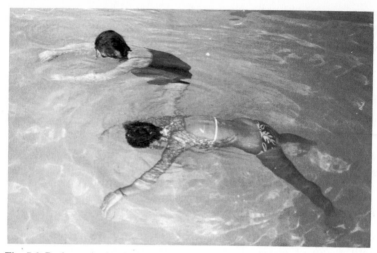

Fig. 7.2 Pool exercise in pregnancy.

how to swim, and they swim this stroke keeping their head high, well above the water. This can be bad for their backs, as lumbar lordosis is unavoidable. The small of the back already needs special attention during pregnancy because of the increased natural curves of the spine, resulting in a more pronounced thoracic cyphosis and lumbar lordosis. In addition the increased body-weight (around 20 to 30 lb towards the end of the pregnancy) adds considerable stress to the intervertebral discs. We have to be very aware of this and should avoid extra strain by working with neck and head in line, thus correcting the lordosis rather than increasing it. However, some exercises cannot be done with the head in line with the spine unless the face is under water, and many women attending either cannot swim or fear water, although they may not admit or realise it. They have to be made gently aware of the fact that as long as air is breathed out through the nose, no water can come in through it. Once they are over this stage, they can learn how to float. The specific weight of the body is slightly higher than the specific weight of water which causes the body to sink. However, if the lungs are full of air, a bigger amount of water is displaced and, applying Archimedes' Law, this means the body experiences a higher upward pressure and will float. Because of the situation of the lungs in the thorax, the body tends to rotate around a transverse axis through the centre of gravity, causing the legs to sink, which is more pronounced if the head is raised out of the water.

This is yet another reason to swim with the head in the water, in order to develop a minimum of resistance (keeping the legs in a horizontal position). It is of utmost importance that the women become aware of the position of their lumbar spine, so that they can constantly correct the hyperlordosis while walking, standing etc. to avoid lower back pain. In addition, awareness of the pelvic floor is an important aspect of these sessions.

b. Relaxation

In the exercises to encourage relaxation, the attention is drawn to the tension in different parts of the body (neck, face, pelvic floor etc.). Once there is an awareness of the tension, relaxation can be learned to relieve it. A series of exercises is designed to help the process. For example, two mothers work together; one mother lies on her back in the water, using floats to keep her legs up. It is not very important which materials are used, as long as the women don't have to squeeze their legs together, for instance by holding a board in between their knees, which is not good preparation for giving birth. In Figure 7.3 the second mother is going to pull the first mother very slowly. With both hands she supports the head, placing her hands behind the ears which are kept below the surface, allowing the head to benefit from the weightlessness. The water also helps to cut off distracting sounds from outside. The mother who is relaxing perceives the movement caused by the turbulence

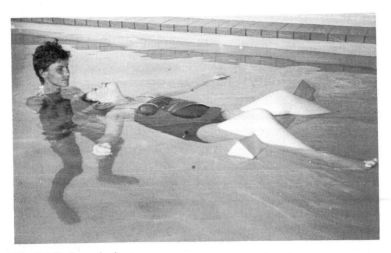

Fig. 7.3 Pool exercise in pregnancy.

of the water as a pleasant micro-massage of the skin. The mother who is doing the pulling has to be inside the water up to her shoulders. If not, she will probably project her shoulders backwards, thus again causing hyperlordosis. If on the contrary she walks backwards pushing back the small of her back, she tilts her pelvis in a corrective position (Fig. 7.3).

c. Gentle shaping up

The purpose of these exercises is to prepare the expectant mother for birth. Since labour and delivery involve important muscle work from the uterus and put extra strain on the cardiovascular and respiratory systems, it seems logical to get the body into shape for this strenuous event. Exercises involving the arms are done, leading towards correcting cyphosis — pulling the shoulders back, bringing the shoulder blades towards the spine and rotating the arms outwards. The arm movement used for the backstroke is very useful for this purpose (Fig. 7.4). The pectoral muscles also get attention, to build up a good supporting base for the breasts which are becoming heavier. Exercises to tone up these muscles should be given in association with corrective exercises for the cyphosis (pulling the shoulders backwards, stretching the upper back), if not the shoulders will be pulled forward. For example, the woman stands up straight, legs forward astride, arms to the sides, holding two floats. She has to bring the floats alternately forwards and backwards, pushing the floats gently down in the water (Figs. 7.5

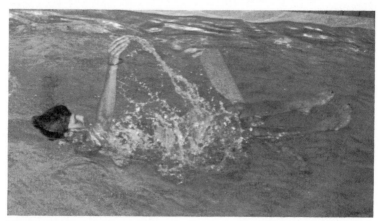

Fig. 7.4 Pool exercise in pregnancy.

and 7.6). In order to correct the changed alignment of the *back*, stretching the back without arching will always be practised: for example, pushing off with two feet at the edge of the pool (ears in between the arms, chin towards the chest), floating out as far as possible, keeping the feet together making it more difficult to keep balance (Fig. 7.7).

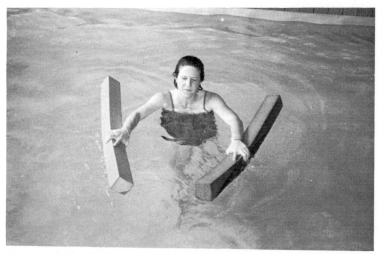

Fig. 7.5 Pool exercise in pregnancy.

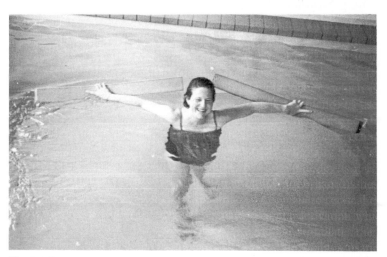

Fig. 7.6 Pool exercise in pregnancy.

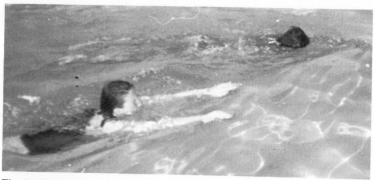

Fig. 7.7 Pool exercise in pregnancy.

Leg work is useful as an attempt to avoid varicose veins. The venous reflow from the legs to the heart is activated by contraction of the muscles surrounding the veins. The blood is squeezed towards the heart whilst a system of valves prevents it from going the wrong way. This system gets obstructed by the weight of the baby pushing upon the veins into the inguinal area in later stages of the pregnancy, thus causing varicose veins. Leg kicks are a very good way to help the blood move towards the heart, and also little jumps. In leg work, it is important not to put too much strain upon the abdominal muscles. For example, holding onto the edge of the pool, lifting up two straight legs, is an exercise to be avoided during pregnancy because the legs meet a lot of resistance from the water. The rectus femoris muscle with attachments to the pelvis contracts, as well as the iliopsoas muscle with insertions on the lumbar vertebrae. As a result of this, the lower back is pulled forwards and the whole pelvis is tilted to the front, causing a hyperlordosis. The abdominal muscles, especially the rectus abdominis, contract to stabilise the pelvis. Contraction of the stretched straight abdominals should never be allowed, especially against resistance, as diastasis can result. A better exercise is the following: the woman lies on her back with two floats under her arms. Whilst breathing out she bends her knees and hips and then bends her head forwards, resulting in a rotation around a transverse axis towards a prone-lying position. She then turns back towards a supine position where inhalation takes place (Figs. 7.8 and 7.9). Her knees must be bent before her head drops back to avoid back-arching and to allow space for the enlarged abdomen; her knees must be apart. An improvement is to have her place the soles

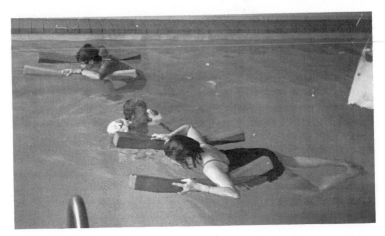

Fig. 7.8 Pool exercise in pregnancy.

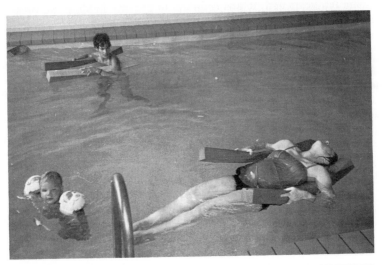

Fig. 7.9 Pool exercise in pregnancy.

of her feet together so that stretching of the inner thigh muscles takes place.

The exercises for the oblique and transverse abdominal muscles are important to help them to withstand the strain of pregnancy and for postnatal recovery. Only by pulling in the abdomen (using the transverse and oblique abdominal fibres) can the woman hope to get her abdomen flat after the birth. These same muscles also play a role during the expulsion of the baby. The ideal is to teach the awareness of the possibility of contracting the upper part and lower part in isolation: the upper part to assist the beginning of the expulsion, the lower part to help towards the end of it. All these muscles are involved in forced expiration. During birth a lot of strain has to be withstood by the muscles of the pelvic floor, especially by the transversus perinei superficialis and profundus, which is why these muscles have to be in good shape. The woman will be asked to alternately contract and release the muscles around vagina and rectum in a lot of different postures. At the same time her body awareness improves, which will be a big help to enable her to release her pelvic floor muscles during birth.

d. Breathing

Some ten years ago, it was common to practise holding the breath as long as possible to encourage pushing throughout the length of the expulsive contraction on a held breath. Water was the ideal place to learn this as with the head submerged it was impossible to breathe in. So our mothers, after a full inhalation, went down, heads under, and got a sound signal every 5 seconds, the aim being to stay under for at least 40 seconds. In the meantime, increasing numbers of obstetricians were encouraging women to breathe through the expulsive process of delivery. In France, Doctor Belaiche (1984) strongly advocates giving birth while blowing out against resistance, involving the oblique and transverse abdominal muscles. He proved how use of the straight abdominal muscles (by active lifting of the head in women giving birth in supine position) causes reflex contraction of the pelvic floor. Because of this revolution, long periods of apnea are now considered to be counter-productive.

Example of a prenatal session

— 5 minutes of gentle swimming.
— Crossing the pool with strides that are as long as possible.
— Jumping forwards, backwards, sideways — changing direction upon a sign.
— Pushing off and floating out as far as possible, arms forward and head in the water, and then swimming the remaining length.
— The same exercise, while exhaling, keeping the two feet well

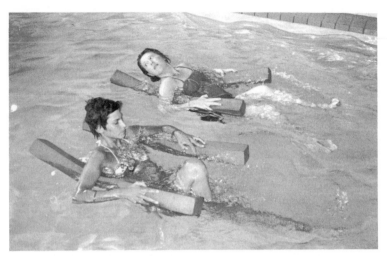

Fig. 7.10 Pool exercise in pregnancy.

together, pulling in the stomach and staying aware of the
position of the small of the back.
— Pushing off again, holding the breath until the speed is lost,
then breathing out quickly through the mouth while releasing
the entire body completely.
— On the back, doing gentle bicycle movements with the legs
(Fig. 7.10).
— Back crawl using arms and legs. In case this is too difficult, the
arms only, supporting the legs by floats.
— Prone-lying: blowing out and releasing, noticing how the body
sinks when the air is gone.
— One foot forwards, one foot backwards, a float under each arm,
joining the two floats alternately in front of and behind the
body, pushing them gently down at the same time.
— Legs astride, arms stretched to the sides, holding floats upon
the water and pushing the two floats far down, keeping the arms
straight.
— Legs astride, keeping the arms with the floats sideways for
balance, bending alternately the left and right knee, thus
shifting the body-weight from left to right, keeping the back
straight and the body on the same level.
— Legs astride, alternately contracting and releasing the pelvic
floor muscles.
— Arms sideways supported by floats, bending the knees while

exhaling, then stretching out the legs to the front (keeping the back vertical). Releasing the legs while inhaling. The legs move down by themselves, supported by the water.

— Arms sideways, supported by floats, bending the knees while exhaling, then stretching out the legs in front. 'Scissoring' the legs slowly, stressing the opening out, then releasing the legs which will sink down on their own, supported by the water.

— Arms sideways, supported by floats, bending the knees while exhaling. Slowly making circles with the feet, keeping the knees stable.

— Supine position, arms sideways supported by floats, bending the knees. Bending the head forwards and rotating forwards towards a prone-lying position while exhaling, without lifting up the legs towards the surface in order to avoid arching. Then first bending the knees, then projecting the head backwards to return to the supine position, inhaling as the face leaves the water.

— Inhaling in supine position. Grasping the knees and releasing. The body will rotate forwards. Then gently inhaling and releasing the pelvic floor while pulling the knees outwards.

— (With a partner): one is holding 2 floats vertically in the water, the back is vertical, the legs are bent and the knees are apart. Holding the floats to the sides while being pulled by the partner. The partner has to pay attention to pushing the small of the back backwards instead of projecting the shoulders backwards and arching the lower back.

— Leg movement of front crawl, holding the head firmly in between both arms.

— Relaxing in supine position, using floats and mats, becoming aware of the breathing (practising abdominal and thoracic breathing with one hand upon the breast, one upon the stomach). Releasing tension, becoming aware of the baby and its movements.

All the exercises have to be executed at the woman's own pace and whenever she feels tired or uncomfortable she should rest or adapt her movements accordingly.

Example of a postnatal session

(The postnatal session is generally more dynamic. More emphasis is laid upon the toning of the abdominal muscles with concentric work, preferably in proximal range, but in fact most of the exercises encompass the total range of movement.)

— Standing astride in a big circle, slowly making big circles with the head without moving the shoulders and trunk.

— Running in a circle with hands joined, singing. On a signal going into prone-lying position, releasing arms and legs and firmly contracting the pelvic floor for as long as possible as the body is carried away by the water.

— Reaching the other side of the pool making little jumps.

— Crossing the pool, walking sideways with big strides, each time reaching as far sideways as possible with one arm (thus side stretching), then reversing the direction.

— Pushing off at the edge and floating out as far as possible and then swimming the remaining length.

— Crossing the pool swimming breast-stroke, with as few strokes as possible, keeping the head and body in line between the strokes.

— Pushing off while breathing out and releasing the entire body.

— Arms sideways supported by floats, lifting up straight legs, keeping the back vertical, then releasing.

— Arms sideways supported by floats, lifting straight legs, opening and closing them, then releasing the legs again.

— Arms sideways supported by floats, lifting straight legs, opening them and letting them float down sideways, then reversing the direction.

— Arms sideways supported by floats, making circles with two straight legs together.

— Contracting and releasing the pelvic floor.

— Legs astride, holding a long float with two hands. Moving the float from one side to the other, pushing it down at the same time.

— Legs astride, arms sideways, pushing floats down with straight arms.

— Grasping the rail, facing the wall, legs apart, toes just below the surface, with little steps and straight legs walking back until the feet are joined, pulling on the arms to stretch the hamstring muscles.

— Supine position, legs supported by floats. Back crawling arm movement.

— In a big circle, every other person in prone-lying position. With the circle moving clockwise, changing from prone-lying to

supine and back. Then the same exercise with the circle moving anti-clockwise.
— All lined up, holding onto floats, a very vigorous crawling leg movement for at least 30 seconds.
— Relaxing upon floats, prolonging the outward breath.

Finally the postnatal session can be followed by baby massage and/or baby swimming.

CONCLUSION

A programme has been developed in France using water as a medium to prepare women physically and mentally for the birth of their babies and the postpartum period. The advantages of this method are numerous: cardiovascular, respiratory, postural, psychological . . . The programme can be offered in any swimming pool with water of a sufficiently high temperature. The ideal is to work as a team in order to exchange different points of view. One of the main goals of the French 'Association Nationale Natation et Maternité' that is now growing to become the International Federation of Perinatal Hydrotherapy, located in Belgium, is to exchange ideas so that there is a continuous evolution and progress towards making the sessions of even greater value.

REFERENCES

Bardiaux M 1984 Statique de la femme enceinte. Equilibre du corps humain. Troubles et modifications de l'équilibre. Les dossiers de l'obstétrique 109: 7–10
Bardiaux M 1984b Indications et contra-indications. Les dossiers de l'obstétrique 109: 15–18
Baum-Sonnenschmidt R 1982 Gebursterleichterung durch Uberwindung Muskslärer Abwehrspannung. Zeitschrift Krankengymnastik 34: 789–795
Belaiche R, Pistre B L'expulsion obstétricale et son préjudice corporal. Unpublished article
Belaiche R 1984 Souffler pour mieux pousser. Enfants magazine 97: 102–105
Delecour M, 1985 La respiration. Unpublished tape-recording. ANNM spring-course. March-Wattignies
Ebersold-Estable E 1984 Le rôle de la sage-femme. Les dossiers de l'obstétrique 109:27
Girardet B 1978 Natation et grossesse. Mémoire pour le C.E.S. de biologie et de médecine du sport. Faculté de médecine Pitié-Salepetrière. Paris VI
Ponsar-Landré M 1985 Apport de la natation au déroulement de la grossesse et de l'accouchement. A l'occasion de deux expériences personnelles. These pour le doctorat en médecine. Faculté de médecine de Bobigny. Paris-Nord
Renner J P 1985 Réflexions sur la poussée expulsive en obstétrique. Le bulletin de l'ANNM. I: 6–8

Two non-pharmacological forms of pain relief in labour

PART 1
ACUPUNCTURE

Irene Skelton

THE USE OF DRUGS FOR PAIN RELIEF IN LABOUR

Most women report labour to be uncomfortable and extremely painful. The pain of labour has been shown to be one of the most severe pains scored using the McGill pain questionnaire (Melzack 1975), with maximum intensity recorded at 8–9 cm cervical dilatation. It seems that the effectiveness of the control of labour pains has not improved over the last twenty years; Beazley (1967) has found that 58% of women questioned reported at least satisfactory levels of analgesia during labour, and a similar survey carried out 15 years later (Morgan et al 1982) showed only 35% reporting a satisfactory level of pain control, and this despite the offer of an epidural block. There is also some concern about the effects of drugs on the neonate. Bupivacaine, used for epidural blocks, crosses the placenta and measurable quantities are found in fetal blood within 10 minutes of administration. Adverse effects on the neonate include increased irritability, decreased motor maturity and muscle tone (Tronick et al 1976). Pethidine, the most commonly used narcotic analgesic, can cause immediate respiratory depression in the baby and can be found in neonate blood up to 6 weeks after delivery with maximum side-effects occurring after 7 days; infants are less alert, more ready to cry and more difficult to quieten (Redshaw and Rosenblatt 1982). Many women who receive pethidine complain of feeling drowsy and disorientated without any decrease of their labour pains. I have recently

129

confirmed this using a visual analogue pain scale to assess pain levels hourly during labour. Of the 30 women who received pethidine, only 5 primigravidae recorded a reduction in pain after administration of the drug and this lasted for up to one hour only (Skelton, unpublished observations). Women are also increasingly concerned about the effects of drugs on their children. A survey I conducted on the third postnatal day of 170 women who delivered in Glasgow Southern General Hospital showed 62% expressing at least some concern with 28% being very concerned (Skelton, in preparation). The general dissatisfaction of many women with the analgesia they receive during labour and the demand for less invasive obstetric practices, has led to an examination of other methods of pain control including acupuncture.

THE HISTORY OF THE USE OF ACUPUNCTURE IN OBSTETRICS

Acupuncture involves the introduction of needles into the skin to help relieve pain and for the treatment of functional illnesses. Traditionally, the needles may be stimulated by manual twirling or by burning herbs attached to the needles. A more recent development has been the use of electro-acupuncture whereby electrodes are attached to selected needles and a stimulus applied in the form of trains of electrical pulses, the parameters of which must be closely controlled and varied depending on the treatment being given. The use of acupuncture to help control labour pain has been used in China and the Far East for many years; mixed reports of its efficacy have been published in Europe, America and the Far East since the early 1970s. Abouleish and Depp (1974) used electro-acupuncture during 12 deliveries. For 7 women the treatment was successful, producing an average of 66% analgesia which was maintained for up to 7.5 h after which conventional analgesia (mainly pethidine) was also used. They concluded that electro-acupuncture was time-consuming, added extra paraphernalia to obstetric procedures and the analgesia produced was incomplete and unpredictable; the women who took part, however, were reported as being delighted with the experiment and would opt for electro-acupuncture for future deliveries. Wallis et al (1974) carried out a study using traditional acupuncture on 21 women and the treatment was unsuccessful in 19 cases. A similar result was reported by Ledergerber (1976) for five deliveries using manually rotated needles, but for 15 deliveries using electro-acupuncture he reported 6 completely successful treatments and 6 complete failures with three partial successes. In Europe, Limoge (1971) and Darras (1974) have reported high levels of success using electro-acupuncture during labour; Kazmie (1985) reported both manual stimulation and electro-acupuncture to be effective in relieving labour pain during 20 deliveries. Electro-acupuncture has been shown to be effective by Hyodo and Gega (1977) in Japan, and Perera (1978) in Sri Lanka. In general, it does seem that electro-acupuncture is more effective than more traditional means of stimulating needles for helping to control labour pain.

TECHNIQUE OF APPLICATION

The most common points used in obstetrics are known as Colon 4, located in the angle at the base of the first and second metacarpals, Stomach 36, located between the heads of the tibia and fibula and Spleen 6 located approximately 10 cm above the internal malleolus on the posterior border of the tibia. Other points which have been used during acupuncture studies and labour pain are located mainly on the midline between the umbilicus and pubis and on the sacrum. These latter and other more peripheral points have been shown to be more effective for the induction and acceleration of labour as opposed to pain control per se (e.g. Theobald 1973, Tsui et al 1977), and are often not practical in the modern management of labour or very beneficial to the comfort or mobility of the women in labour. I have found Colon 4 is also impractical and restricting, especially when an intravenous infusion is also required. Needling points on the sacrum is obviously a great hindrance to movement. Electro-acupuncture in close proximity to the uterus should be avoided because the possibility of electrical interference with the recording of fetal heart rate has been reported by Abouleish and Depp (1975). There is also the possibility of secondary fetal distress due to tetanic uterine contraction.

In the author's experience, sufficient levels of analgesia can be achieved using electro-acupuncture on two leg points only, usually Spleen 6 and Neima, a point located approximately half-way between the head of the tibia and the internal malleolus which, in the Chinese literature, is said to provide analgesia for abdominal and pelvic surgery. For particularly anxious women, I have found the points Stomach 36 and Neima to be especially effective during the early stages of labour, with Neima and Spleen 6 used after cervical dilatation has reached 5–6 cm. It is sufficient to use only one leg, thereby minimising interference with usual obstetric practices and the women's movements.

AURICULAR ACUPUNCTURE

The use of auricular acupuncture points, found in the concha and on both lateral and medial aspects of the pinna, and which are thought to correspond to specific parts of the body, is often the first choice treatment by many acupuncture practitioners for the control of acute pain (Fig. 8.1). However, there is little published information on the use of auricular acupuncture in the control of labour pain, although the effect of needling ear points on cervical dilatation has been reported (Heyuan and Lithua 1984). Kazmie (1985) has reported the use of auricular points in the later stages of labour. Auricular correspondence points which should be needled are indicated as areas of increased electrical conductance compared to the adjacent skin, and can be located using an appropriate electrical meter. They are often tender and can also be located by palpation with a blunt probe. In the author's experience, areas corresponding to the uterus, bladder and sciatic region are the main points which become active during labour, although there are others. These were needled and a press pin, rather like a small drawing pin or thumb tack and offering minimum interference, left in situ covered by a piece of Opsite or Micropore for the duration of the labour. The bladder correspondence point should not be used for induced labours because of the possibility of tetanic contractions of the uterus and fetal distress. The bladder meridian is one amongst

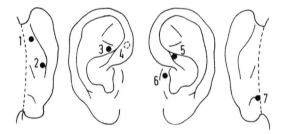

1. Low Back	5. Bladder
2. Shoulder	6. Conception Vessel
3. Sciatic	Governor Vessel
4. Uterus	7. Sympathetic

Fig. 8.1 Auricular acupuncture points.

others which is described in texts on traditional acupuncture as being used for induction and also for abortion. The use of these meridians is to be avoided when treating women with acupuncture during the antenatal period.

STUDY AT THE SOUTHERN GENERAL HOSPITAL, GLASGOW

In the light of increasing dissatisfaction expressed by an increasing number of women in the use of drugs during childbirth and the mixed results which have been reported using acupuncture, I have re-assessed the effectiveness of electro-acupuncture compared to conventional methods of controlling labour pain (Skelton in preparation). The study involved 170 deliveries over a period of two years at the Southern General Hospital, Glasgow. Assessing pain is extremely difficult because of the high subjective element. Most methods have been designed to assess chronic as opposed to the acute pain with increasing intensity characteristic of labour. In a pilot to the main study, I used a visual analogue scale to assess pain during labour. This method avoids the use of numbers and descriptors, thereby reducing both suggestability and attention on the pain; it was found to be readily understood by the participating women and did not intrude with any relaxation techniques being used during labour. Revill et al (1976) have taken hourly mean analogue pain scores during labour and found that the increase closely paralleled cervical dilatation, and the method has been shown to be reasonably sensitive for the measurement of severe pain (Rosen 1979). For these reasons, I opted for the use of a visual analogue pain scale in the main study to assess pain during labour.

Labour pain has been shown to be influenced by a complex interaction between fear, anxiety, age, menstrual history, parity, family background, cultural and socio-economic considerations. A great deal of the fear and anxiety regarding labour can be relieved by antenatal preparation and psychoprophylaxis. Because of this complex interaction, consideration was given to emotional and muscular tension levels exhibited by women taking part in the study prior to delivery, as well as social class and attendance of antenatal preparation classes. Two groups of 85 women, matched for age, parity and social class, received either electro-acupuncture or conventional analgesia, including epidural block, during labour. In the acupuncture group, 37 received additional analgesia and were treated as a separate group designated acupuncture-plus. Of

Table 8.1. Mean highest pain scores (HPS± standard error) recorded during labour using an analogue pain scale

Group	N	HPS	Parity	N	HPS
Control	83	76.0 ± 2.2	Primigravida	33	77.3 ± 3.8
			Multipara	50	73.8 ± 2.8
Acupuncture	48	57.3 ± 2.7	Primigravida	9	65.4 ± 4.7
			Multipara	39	55.7 ± 3.0
Acupuncture plus	35	77.0 ± 2.8	Primigravida	25	80.0 ± 3.0
			Multipara	10	74.7 ± 6.5

The mean pain score for the multipara was significantly less than that for primigravidae (F = 9.600, 1 × 164 d.f., P < 0.05). In the acupuncture group, the primigravidae recorded a lower mean pain score than the acupuncture-plus group (F = 6.069, 1 × 32 d.f., P < 0.05), and the score for the multipara was significantly lower than both the control group (F = 18.670, 1 × 87 d.f., P < 0.05) and acupuncture-plus group, (F = 7.698, 1 × 47 d.f., P < 0.05). No significant difference was found between the control and acupuncture-plus groups (F = 0.455, 1 × 117 d.f., P = not significant).

these, only 10 reported inadequate analgesia with acupuncture, 8 were extremely distressed on admission, 18 developed unforeseen complications during labour and there was equipment failure during one delivery. Muscle and emotional scores were assessed using the Crawford method designed for use by midwives during labour (Meissner 1980).

The mean highest pain score recorded during labour for the primigravidae was found to be significantly higher than for the multiparous women (see Table 8.1). The scores were significantly lower for the primigravidae in the acupuncture group compared to the acupuncture-plus group, and lower than both the control and acupuncture-plus groups for the multiparous women. Since the participating women could leave the acupuncture group at any stage in the study, it could be argued that the lower scores in that group could be attributed to women with the most pain opting out of the group during labour. However, there was no significant difference between those leaving the acupuncture group during labour, the acupuncture-plus group and the control group, suggesting this not to be the case. There were no significant differences between the groups in muscle or emotional tension scores, and no significant differences were found in tension scores between attenders and non-attenders of antenatal classes. However, the mean highest pain score recorded during labour was lower for the attenders. There was no significant difference in Apgar scores between the three groups.

It has been suggested that acupuncture can decrease blood loss and the duration of labour (Perera 1978). For spontaneous, unaug-

Table 8.2. Mean length of labour with spontaneous onset (hours standard error) and estimated blood loss (ml standard error).

Group	N	First stage (Hours SE)	Second stage (Hours SE)	Estimated Blood Loss (ml SE)
Control				
Primigravida	14	9.7 ± 0.7	1.4 ± 0.2	177 ± 19
Multipara	26	6.2 ± 0.6	0.5 ± 0.1	219 ± 21
Acupuncture				
Primigravida	8	7.2 ± 1.0	1.0 ± 0.2	125 ± 25
Multipara	22	6.5 ± 0.6	0.4 ± 0.1	177 ± 27
Acupuncture plus				
Primigravida	7	9.1 ± 0.1	1.0 ± 0.2	241 ± 89
Multipara	2	9.4 ± 4.0	0.4 ± 0.2	150 ± 50

The duration of the first stage of labour was significantly shorter for the primigravidae in the acupuncture group compared to controls ($t = 2.121$, 20 d.f., $P < 0.05$).

No significant difference in estimated loss of blood was found ($F = 1.212$, 5×71 d.f., P = not significant).

mented labours (Table 8.2), the first stage was found to be significantly shorter for the primigravidae in the acupuncture group. Kazmie (1985) has also reported shorter labours using acupuncture. These data suggest that acupuncture has a very positive contribution to make, both for pain control during labour and other considerations such as duration, particularly for primigravidae. There was no indication in the Glasgow study that acupuncture decreased estimated blood loss during labour.

A striking feature of the use of acupuncture which was consistently reported by women in the study who delivered under acupuncture, was the feeling of calm, 'well-being', and control they were able to maintain over their labour, the very features which are often reported as being absent during deliveries using conventional analgesics. These observations were especially relevant when reported by multiparous women who had previous deliveries with which to compare their experiences with acupuncture. A survey carried out as part of the main study on the third postnatal day showed 83% of the acupuncture group were 'very satisfied' with the feeling of control over their labour as opposed to 53% in the control group. This response was reflected in answers to the question 'Were you satisfied with the method of analgesia used?', with 72% of the acupuncture group recording 'very much' satisfaction compared with 41% of the control group (31% for those who received pethidine alone).

The procedures developed for the Glasgow study involved the

use of few needles, just two points on one leg attached to wires from an electro-acupuncture unit and small, semi-permanent press pins in one or two auricular acupuncture points. The needles used in the legs were made of 32 gauge stainless steel and bent at right-angles at about 5 mm from the point so that, once inserted, they could be taped to the skin with electrodes attached to minimise the risk of being dislodged during labour. It was found that electro-acupuncture should be commenced before cervical dilatation reaches 4 cm. However, satisfactory levels of analgesia were achieved when electro-acupuncture was commenced as late as 7 cm dilatation with multiparous women. For induced labours, needles were introduced 1–2 hours after induction. Electro-acupuncture was initiated with the electro-acupuncture unit set at a frequency of 2.5 Hz at an intensity just below the maximum tolerance threshold, and the women were invited to control the frequency but not the intensity of stimulation. Most women gradually increased the frequency to the maximum allowed by the unit of 80 Hz by the time cervical dilatation had reached 7–8 cm. Stimulation was maintained until delivery and, if the perineum was damaged, continued until the necessary repairs had been carried out. Many women experienced much discomfort when the frequency was set at 20 Hz. This observation was regularly and consistently reported by staff in the labour suite and it is recommended that this frequency is avoided.

DISCUSSION

Several different models have been advanced explaining how acupuncture might work, and limited space does not allow a full exposition. That which is probably most relevant to pain control during labour is the biochemical model involving the neuropeptides. The best known neuropeptides, certainly in the area of pain control, are the opioid peptides, the endorphins and the enkephalins. The discovery of opiate peptide binding sites in the central nervous system during the early 1970s, led to the anticipation of a specific role for neuropeptides in pain control. Subsequent investigations on the distribution of the receptor sites and the proliferation in the number of different active opioids to 18 or more, not all with analgesic properties, have increased the range of functions in which they seem to be involved to include the immune and the endocrine systems as well as emotion and behaviour (e.g. see Pert et al 1985). The 'endorphin effect' has been taken by some as being *the* mechanism to explain how acupuncture might work, and research on the biochemical changes associated with acupuncture, in particular electro-acupuncture, has concentrated on the opioid peptides. The number of papers identifying the involvement of endorphins and enkephalins in acupuncture has mushroomed since the original studies in the mid-1970s (e.g. Mayer 1975, Pomeranz and Chui 1976, Sjolund et al 1977).

The implication of the opioid peptides in pain control using acupuncture has been based, to a large extent, on the reversal of analgesia when the drug naloxone, an antagonist to opiates, is administered. However, some caution should be exercised when interpreting results based only on inhibition by naloxone, since its action is not specific to opiates (Hayes et al 1977) and the literature contains an apparently bewildering mixture of conflicting results involving naloxone inhibition (e.g. see Woolf and Wall 1983). More direct evidence comes from measured increases in opioid concentrations in the cerebro-spinal fluid (e.g. Clement-Jones et al 1980), in blood plasma (e.g. Nappi et al 1982) and from studies using antibodies specific to each peptide (e.g. Han et al 1984). There is evidence that the characteristics of analgesia produced using electro-acupuncture can depend on the frequency of the stimulation (Anderson et al 1973), with 2 Hz producing a more generalised effect but of shorter duration compared with 10–100 Hz. Subsequent work has shown that two analgesic mechanisms may be working during electro-acupuncture. Analgesia produced at below 10–15 Hz can be inhibited by naloxone implicating the opioid peptides, and that produced at frequencies greater than around 100 Hz can be at least partially inhibited by ρ-chlorophenylanaline, an antagonist to the monoamine neurotransmitter, 5-hydroxytryptamine (5-HT or serotonin), and by the destruction of the raphe nucleus, a region of the brain which is a rich store of 5-HT (McLennan 1977, Cheng and Pomeranz 1979, 1981). Acupuncture analgesia has been demonstrated to increase or decrease in proportion with 5-HT levels in the central nervous system (Han et al 1979). Thus it seems that at frequencies less than around 10 Hz, opioid peptides are dominant in the analgesic mechanism, and at higher frequencies, 5-HT predominates. It should be remembered that there is much conflicting evidence about the role of various active agents in acupuncture analgesia, and much of it comes from experimental animals where reactions to painful stimuli are used to infer a relationship between pain and the stimulus which might be untenable. However, it is interesting to note the author's

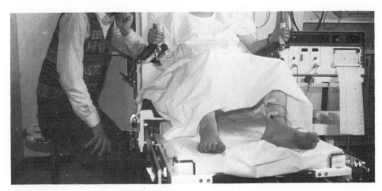

Fig. 8.2

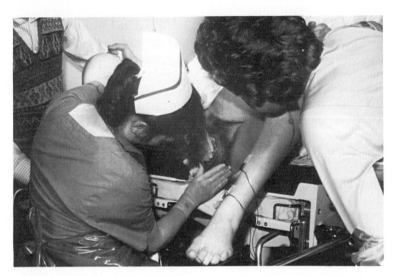

Fig. 8.3

Fig. 8.2 and 8.3 Acupuncture in the second stage of labour — two leg points in use.

experience that women in labour using electro-acupuncture gradually increase the frequency of the stimulation from 2.5 Hz to the maximum possible during the course of their labour, and it is tempting to suggest that maximum use of both possible analgesic mechanisms is being employed. This can only be confirmed by extensive pharmacological investigations during labour (Figs. 8.2 and 8.3).

CONCLUSION

In conclusion, the author considers that electro-acupuncture, appropriately used, can make a significant contribution to the control of pain during labour. The factors underlying labour pain are very complex (e.g. see Melzack 1984), and the search for methods of relieving the intense pain of labour is the lot of the midwife, obstetrician, anaesthetist and physiotherapist. No one method reduces pain and at the same time leaves the woman satisfied and fulfilled by her experiences of childbirth. The work of Morgan and colleagues (1982) shows that lower levels of pain do not necessarily give rise to high levels of satisfaction. My own work shows that there is a place for acupuncture in the control of labour pain and that its use gives a greater level of satisfaction with the experiences of childbirth than conventional analgesics, especially pethidine. A major problem is the lack of availability of the therapy, a problem which can be overcome by more midwives and physiotherapists undertaking suitable training and practising acupuncture, not only for the control of labour pain, but also for the treatment of many of the complaints which accompany pregnancy and the postnatal period. The World Health Organization sees the wealth of information favouring acupuncture as undeniable evidence that the therapy should be considered as an important element in primary health care, fully integrated with conventional medicine, and that includes obstetrics.

ACKNOWLEDGEMENT

I gratefully acknowledge the help of M. W. Flowerdew PhD, Research Adviser to The International Society of Biophysical Medicine, 18 Water Street, Liverpool L2 8TD, UK in writing this contribution.

REFERENCES

Abouleish E, Depp R 1975 Acupuncture in obstetrics. Anaesthesia and Analgesia 51: 1–83
Anderson S A, Eriksson T, Holmgren E et al 1973 Electro-acupuncture: effect on pain threshold measured with electrical stimulation of teeth. Brain Research 63: 393–396
Beazley J M 1967 Relief of pain in labour. The Lancet 2: 1033–1035
Cheng R S S, Pomeranz B 1979 Electro-acupuncture analgesia could be mediated by two pain-relieving mechanisms: endorphin and non-endorphin systems. Life Sciences 25: 1957–1962

Cheng R S S, Pomeranz B 1981 Monoaminergic mechanisms of electro-acupuncture analgesia. Brain Research 215: 77–92

Clement-Jones V V, McLoughlin L, Tomlin S et al 1980 Increased β-endorphin but not met-enkephalin levels in human cerebro-spinal fluid after acupuncture for recurrent pain. The Lancet 2: 946–949

Darras J C 1974 Acupuncture Update 1974. Report on a Symposium held by the National Acupuncture Research Society, New York

Han C-S, Chou P-H, Lu C-C et al 1979 The role of central 5-HT in acupuncture analgesia. Scientia Sinica 22: 91–104

Han J-S, Xie G-A, Zhou Z-J et al 1984 Acupuncture mechanisms in rabbits; studies in microinjection of antibodies against β-endorphin, enkephalin and substance P. Neuropharmacology 23: 1–6

Hayes R, Price D D, Dubner R 1977 Naxolone antagonism as evidence for narcotic mechanisms. Science, Washington D. C. 196:600

Heyuan Z, Lithua Y 1984 Observations on the effect of auriculo-acupuncture for dilatation of cervix in 56 cases. Abstract 87 in Second National Symposium on Acupuncture and Moxibustion and Acupuncture Anaesthesia. The Peoples' Medical Publishing House, Beijing

Hyodo M, Gega O 1977 Use of acupuncture anaesthesia for normal delivery. American Journal of Chinese Medicine 5: 63–69

Kazmie M 1985 Acupuncture analgesia in obstetrics. 1st International Symposium on Acupuncture and Electro-Therapeutics, October 1985, New York. Acupuncture and Electro-therapeutics Research 10(3): 233

Ledergerber C P 1976 Electro-acupuncture in obstetrics. Acupuncture and Electro-therapeutics Research 2: 105–111

Limoge A 1971 Obstetric Electroanalgesia. In: Nervous System and Electric Currents. II. Plenum Press, New York, pp 189–193

Mayer D J 1975 Opiate receptor mechanisms. Neurosci Res Prog Bull 13: 98

McLennan H, Gifilla K, Heap Y 1977 Some pharmacological observations on the analgesia induced by acupuncture in rabbits. Pain 3: 229–238

Meissner J E 1980 Predicting a patient's anxiety level during labour. Nursing (USA) July 1980, 50–51

Melzack R 1975 The McGill Pain Questionnaire: major properties and scoring methods. Pain 1: 277–299

Melzack R 1984 The myth of painless childbirth. Pain 19: 321–337

Morgan B, Bulpitt C J, Clifton P, Lewis P J 1982 Effectiveness of pain relief in labour —survey of 1000 mothers. British Medical Journal 285: 689–690

Nappi G, Facchine F, Bono G et al 1982 Plasma levels in post-traumatic chronic headache and trigeminal neuralgia: maintained responses to acupuncture. Headache 22: 276–279

Perera W 1978 Acupuncture in childbirth. International Symposium, Sri Lanka, 1978

Pert C, Ruff M R, Weber R J, Herkenham M 1985 Neuropeptides and their receptors: a psychosomatic network. Journal of Immunology 135 (2): 820s–826s

Pomeranz B, Chui D 1976 Naxolone blockade of acupuncture analgesia: endorphin implicated. Life Sciences 19: 1757–1762

Redshaw M, Rosenblatt D B 1982 The influence of analgesia in labour on the baby. Midwife Health Visitor Community Nurse 18: 126–132

Revill S I, Robinson J O, Rosen M, Hogg M I J 1976 The reliability of a linear analogue scale of evaluating pain. Anaesthesia 31: 1198

Rosen M 1979 Systematic and inhalation analgesia. British Journal of Anaesthesia 51: p. 115

Sjolund B, Terenius L, Eriksson M 1977 Increased cerebro-spinal fluid levels of endorphin after electro-acupuncture. Acta Physiologica Scandinavica 100: 382–384

Theobald G W 1973 The Electrical Stimulation of Labour. Butterworth, London

Tronick E, Wise S, Als H, Adamson L, Scanlon J, Brazelton T B 1976 Regional obstetric anaesthesia and newborn behaviour: effect over the first ten days of life. Paediatrics 58: 94–100

Tsui J J, Lai Y F, Sharma S D 1977 The influence of acupuncture stimulation during pregnancy. Obstetrics and Gynecology 50: 479–488

Wallis I, Schnider S M, Palahnuik R J et al 1974 An investigation of acupuncture analgesia in obstetrics. Anaesthesiology 6: 596–604

Woolf C J, Wall P D 1983 Endogenous opioid peptides and pain mechanisms: a complex relationship. Nature (London) 306, 739–740

PART 2
TRANSCUTANEOUS ELECTRICAL NERVE STIMULATION

Janette Krzyszton

INTRODUCTION

Obstetric physiotherapy has vastly improved in recent years with pre- and postnatal education programmes preparing women and their partners for their role as parents (Barlow et al 1978). The physiotherapist should be conversant with the latest techniques and procedures available in order to provide positive health care education.

In the 1970s the urge for more natural methods of birthing increased. The concern about side-effects of drugs used in labour became widespread, and in some birth centres alternatives to analgesia drugs were offered.

HISTORY OF TENS USE IN LABOUR

One of the methods used was transcutaneous electrical nerve stimulation (TENS), first reported in 1971 by Persaninov et al in Russia. In 1974, Shealy et al in the USA found excellent control of posterior pain in 50 labouring women, but only 10% of anterior pain was relieved. In 1977, Augustinsson et al used TENS for 147 parturients with 48% perceiving good relief, 37% some relief and the rest only minimal. In 1979, Stewart found the results summarised in Figure 8.4.

In 1980, Erkkola, Pikkola and Kanto used TENS in 100 vaginally delivered women compared with 100 who used conventional drugs (see Table 8.3). 31% of the TENS group reported good pain relief; 55% reported moderate relief. In 1981, Bundsen, Peterson

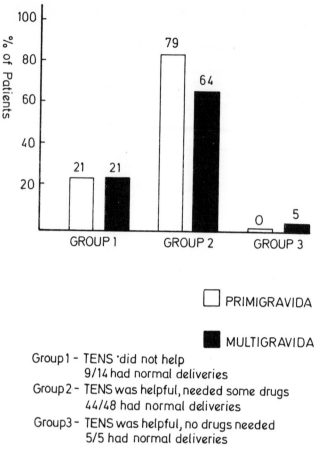

Fig. 8.4 Evaluation of analgesic need in TENS treated women in labour.

and Selstam reviewed 566 vaginally delivered women randomly assigned to TENS or conventional analgesia. TENS reduced stage one pain, but intense suprapubic pain was unrelieved in the majority. In 1982, 24 women who were being induced (usually because of pre-eclampsia or post-term pregnancy) were studied (along with a control group) using TENS in labour by Bundsen, Ericson, Peterson and Thiringer. In first stage, low back pain was reduced in the TENS group; in transition, suprapubic pain was not altered to any great degree in either group; and of the 15 who proceeded to second stage, 8 reported good analgesia in the TENS group.

Table 8.3 Subjective evaluation of TENS benefit (n = 100) (Based on the study by Erkkola et al, 1980)

Pain relief	Mother	Midwife
Good	31	40
Moderate	55	50
None	14	10

$X^2 = 2.0$ not significantly different

In 1983, a study by Merry using a non-functional placebo unit and a functional TENS unit, on 17 women, failed to show any significant difference between the two groups. A visual analogue scale of pain was used before and after 30 to 60 minutes of use of TENS; so whether the relatively brief period of subjective pain assessment after initiating TENS was not an adequate representation, it is difficult to comment on. In 1986 a study was initiated in Sydney, but no preliminary data is available. There are many other studies, but a cross-section has been cited above.

TENS AS A MODALITY

TENS as a pain control modality was originally reported in the early days of Rome and Greece when live torpedo fish and electric fish organs were placed on 'patients' (Taub and Kane 1975). Galvanic generators were the next step in the 1800s (Green 1953), used by mainly non-medical operators. In 1965 Melzack and Wall resurrected interest in electrical neuro-modulation as a non-invasive pain treatment. Their gate theory of pain provided a scientific basis for the use of TENS. In the late 1960s Doctor Shealy used TENS to screen dorsal column stimulator recipients. He noted that the TENS often afforded adequate analgesia without the need for further invasive procedures. Since that time it has been used successfully for both acute and chronic pain (Lampe 1978).

USES OF TENS IN LABOUR

By 1986 there were many models of TENS units available. For obstetrical usage the dual channel systems are most efficacious, as the C and A delta mediated types of pain occur at different times in the labour and from T10 to S4 areas (see Fig. 8.5) which are too vast for effective use of just one channel. The units are small,

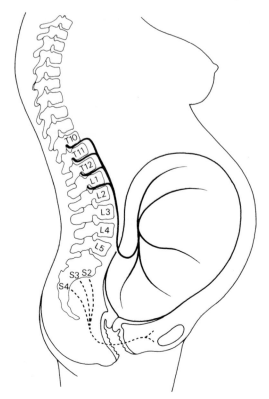

Fig. 8.5 Sketch depicting innervation of pain of parturition.

light and battery operated. The stimulator delivers electrical impulses through the skin which bombards the brain with comfortable afferent impulses. Each channel has separate controls for output, pulse width and rate to allow precise adjustment during various stages of labour. Models available in Australia have outputs from 0–100 mA, voltage up to 160 V, frequency of 10–300 pulses per second and duration of 10–500 microsecs (adapted from Wadsworth et al 1979). They produce either square or spiked biphasic wave forms which have prime action on sensory nerves at the outputs used for analgesia.

The models investigated for this review include the Microceptor II (used in an unpublished pilot study in 1979 in Sydney), Q.B. TENS (used in Brisbane in 1984–1986 in unpublished studies), and 3M Tenzcare (used in 1986 in Sydney for an ongoing study).

The comparisons have been collated for reference in Table 8.4.

Table 8.4

	Microceptor II	Q. B. TENS	3 M Tenzcare
Model	Now replaced by 'Orion' model Dual channel	Dual channel	Dual channel with patient hand control to increase output
Electrodes	Round or long carbon	Round carbon	Long self-adhesive or carbon with gel and tape
Test load	510 ohms	510 ohms	510 ohms
Amplitude	0–160 V peak	0–32 V peak	0–32 V peak
Pulse width	10 microsecs	350 microsecs	20–225microsecs
Frequency	11–100 HZ	15–166 HZ	10–200 HZ
Wave form	Biphasic spiked wave	Balanced biphasic square wave	Balanced biphasic square wave
Supplier	CIG Medishield Sydney	W G Medbury Sydney	3M Australia Sydney
Batteries	Rechargeable	Rechargeable	Rechargeable
Rechargers	Supplied with unit	Supplied with unit	Supplied with unit

For labour, rechargeable batteries are vital as their lifetime is approximately 12 hours if well charged initially, and obviously they may be required for longer periods in the parturient. It should be noted that analgesia is less effective once the batteries are reducing in output, so spare charged batteries should be on hand at all times. Long (12 cm) electrodes allow one application, i.e. from T10–L1 and S2–S4 at the beginning of labour, without the need to change electrode positions while labour is progressing. (Fig. 8.6). This causes less interruption to ongoing nursing and monitoring of the labour, which is an important factor in gaining labour ward staff acceptance of use of the unit. They can either be self-adhesive, hypoallergenic, conductive electrodes, or carbon electrodes applied with hypoallergenic gel and taped onto the appropriate level paravertebrally with skin tape. Each pair conducts a current across the spine levels it is placed at, thus interfering with the pain stimuli from organs/tissues innervated by the same nerves. Thus in stage one, where cervical distention, stretching and tearing causes pain receptor activation which is mediated by unmyelinated C fibres, the mother stimulates the T10–L1 paraspinal areas on her back and blocks the pain sensation with the 'pins and needles' sensation from the TENS machine.

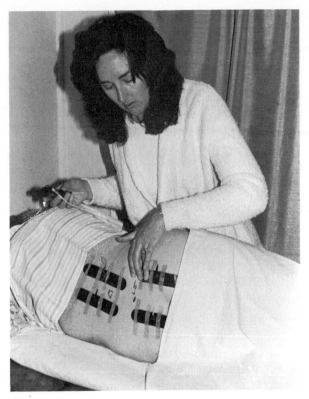

Fig. 8.6 Author applying electrodes.

In 'transition', and second stage, when sharper (myelinated A delta) pain is perceived from stretching, tearing and possible haemorrhage of fascia, skin, subcutaneous tissues and other pain sensitive structures, the second current can be added at S2–S4 to reduce the sensations perceived from these areas. If the above usual placements are not effective, other sites can be tried, e.g. thoracic levels to influence sympathetic nerves, or over the abdomen. It is not fully understood how TENS works at the intraspinal or brain level, but release of local or distant neurotransmitters is the most likely factor.

ANTENATAL INSTRUCTION

The idea of TENS should be mooted in antenatal classes and interested couples encouraged to seek obstetrician consent for its use. The obstetrician should be informed as fully as possible about TENS by the physiotherapist. The hospital to be attended should be contacted if they do not already have an ongoing TENS programme. The labour ward staff must be happy to have the couple using the machine or its use will be abandoned due to lack of encouragement.

Thus, the first step is public relations in ensuring all involved people are happy to use it. In a home birth situation, the midwife or physiotherapist may actually bring the machine and attach the electrodes, rather than the hospital ward staff or physiotherapist on call being involved when the labouring woman comes into hospital.

The machine should be discussed, electrode placement shown and a trial use on the woman's arm undertaken during classes. The settings she tends to find most comfortable should be documented to facilitate TENS early use in labour. An informed consent form should be signed, as is usual in any hospital admission, but specifically for use of TENS. The visual analogue scale should be demonstrated so that its use for documenting pain in labour will be made easier. It is a 10 cm line beginning on the left with 'zero pain' and on the right ending with 'maximum pain'. The woman should document her pain on admission to hospital and then at regular intervals, e.g. fifteen minutes for 2–3 hours, then $\frac{1}{2}$ hourly or hourly until 'transition' and second and third stages are complete. This scale of pain is used to determine the efficacy of analgesia and record data for future use, but is not vital to the use of TENS, obviously. A hand-out on the rationale behind TENS and its use in labour should be given to the participating couple during their antenatal training, and questions invited. These should be answered with the degree of technical detail required by the individuals. A contact telephone number with a physiotherapist, obstetrician or local doctor conversant with the unit should be available for discussion of TENS and any other queries the couple might have. Translations in various languages would assist compliance in cases where a knowledgeable interpreter is not available.

The positive aspects of TENS usage should be emphasised to the user. Any labouring postures may be employed, e.g. standing and walking in first stage, prone in bean bag, and various modified sitting to four-point kneeling positions as shown in classes (Fig. 8.7). The relaxation and visualisation techniques practised in classes can be better concentrated on with TENS reducing the level

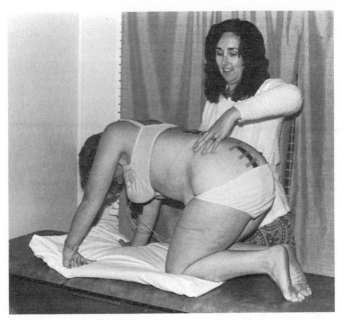

Fig. 8.7 Author encouraging pelvic rocking with electrodes in situ.

of pain. Therefore, concentration on and enjoyment of parturition is facilitated. A comfortable tingling is felt, which is increased as each contraction builds up, then is reduced to a mild sensation as the contraction fades. Any other medical intervention is possible while using TENS. Usually the need for extra medication is reduced in TENS users (Bundsen et al 1981, 1982). Neonatal condition in these studies was somewhat better in the TENS group compared with controls, and other studies have shown no differences.

In all studies of Apgar scores, TENS groups do well. Ultrasound monitoring is not interfered with by TENS. Some interference with fetal heart monitoring may occur with TENS usage, so Bundsen developed an artefact suppression filter which removes the effect of TENS on the electrocardiogram of the fetus. The main advantage of its use is that stage 1 pain is markedly reduced, allowing the parturient to play a more active, alert part in the process she is undergoing. Since suprapubic pain is not much reduced by any type of pain relief including TENS, non-drug methods are preferable. The woman has control over the analgesic modality, and this lessens her feeling of dependence in an inexorable situation which could otherwise leave her feeling helpless and in the complete control of others. Last but not least, TENS could possibly shorten labour if pain is less and relaxation is facilitated to encourage the expulsion of the fetus.

The role of the partner in TENS usage is to support the woman in its use and, in some hospitals, to apply electrodes. The importance of partner presence is not lessened, and in fact communication is improved as the woman is not 'phased out' because of medications. They can better share the joy of their new experience if both can take an active part in the birthing process. As is usual in antenatal classes, the factors influencing pain of labour and delivery should be mentioned to the pregnant woman, i.e. size of fetus, gestational age, presentation of fetus, size of mother's pelvis, parity, strength of contractions, sleep deprivation effects, attitude and mood of parturient, prior experience of pain, personality, ethnic and cultural patterns, anxiety and motivation.

The only contra-indications to TENS, applicable to labour, are the parturient's use of demand cardiac pacemaker or worsening pain.

CONCLUSION

Often simple solutions are disregarded when age old problems arise. Delivering a baby is perhaps the oldest 'age old problem' and TENS is a simple solution. The propagation of its use in labour depends on how it is presented to traditional birthing supporters, i.e. doctors, midwives and labour ward staff. The evidence is mounting to prove its safety and efficacy, and physiotherapists should use every opportunity to communicate the simplicity, cost effectiveness, safety and proven results of TENS to those who can establish its widespread availability.

ACKNOWLEDGEMENT

I would like to convey my thanks to Bruce Roberts at 3M in Sydney, who conducted the oscilloscope studies on the three machines included in the review.

REFERENCES

Augustinsson L E, Bohlin P, Bundsen P, Carlsson C A, Forssman L, Sjoberg P, Tyreman N O 1977 Pain relief during delivery by transcutaneous electrical nerve stimulation. Pain 4: 59–65

Barlow B, Colgan A, Cox J 1978 The work of the Obstetric Physiotherapist. Physiotherapy 64:8 229–230

Bundsen P, Peterson L E, Selstam U 1981 Pain relief in labour by transcutaneous electrical nerve stimulation: A prospective matched study. Acta Obstetrica et Gynecologica Scandinavica 60: 459–468

Bundsen P, Ericson K, Peterson L E, Thiringer K 1982 Pain relief in labour by TENS: Testing of a modified stimulation technique and evaluation of the neurological and biochemical condition of the newborn infant. Acta Obstetrica et Gynecologica Scandinavica 61: 129–136

Erkkola R, Pikkola P, Kanto J 1980 Transcutaneous nerve stimulation for pain relief during labour. A controlled study. Annales Chirurgiae et Gynaecologiae 69: 273–277

Green R 1953 Galvani: commentary on electricity. Elizabeth Licht, Publisher, Cambridge MA

Lampe G 1978 Introduction to the use of TENS devices. Physical Therapy 58:12 1450–1454

Melzack R, Wall P 1965 Pain mechanisms: a new theory. Science 150:3699 971–979

Merry A F 1983 Use of TENS in labour. New Zealand Medical Journal 96: 635–638

Persaninov L, Kastrubin E 1971 Use of therapeutic analgesia with impulse currents during labour. Sovetskaia Meditsina 34:10 32–35.

Shealy C, Maurer D 1974 TENS for control of pain Surgical Neurology 2: 45–47

Stewart P 1979 Transcutaneous nerve stimulaton as a method of analgesia in labour. Anesthesia 34: 361–364

Taub A, Kane K 1975 A history of local analgesia Pain 1: 125–138

Wadsworth H, Chanmugam A 1979 Electrophysical Agents in Physiotherapy. Science Press, Australia

Urinary incontinence and the pelvic floor

INTRODUCTION

The physiotherapist has been associated with the treatment of various gynaecological conditions in women, including urinary incontinence, for many years. Textbooks from the past discuss the use of baths, douches, light, ionisation and various forms of heat to assist in the management of these conditions. Green Armytage (1948) presented a lecture to the British Congress of Obstetrics and Gynaecology entitled 'The role of physiotherapy in Obstetrics and Gynaecology'. He mentioned that 30 years earlier Stacey Wilson in Birmingham first advocated the use of pelvic exercises in 'hyposthenic' girls showing signs of congenital prolapse, incontinence and backache. Also, he reported that his colleagues in France stated that with exercise the muscles of the pelvic floor could be strengthened sufficiently to 'casser une noisette'!

Arnold Kegel (1949) in California was an early protagonist of conservative management for urinary incontinence. He published an article on 'The Physiologic Treatment of Poor Tone and Function of the Genital muscles and of Urinary Stress Incontinence'. He commented that between 30% and 40% of women lack the normal function of the perineal muscles.

Prevalence

Incontinence is defined as wanting in self-restraint or acting without restraint, and may be applied to secrets, tongue, urine or faeces. The International Continence Society (1977) has recommended the following definition when this term is used in reference to urinary incontinence — 'A condition in which involuntary loss of urine is a social or hygienic problem and is objectively demonstrable.'

During recent years there has been increasing interest in diagnosing and treating this condition. This is timely since it is a common problem and, as the average age of the population rises, it will occur with greater frequency unless we explore ways to promote continence and improve our methods of managing uncontrollable urinary leakage. Currently one in three women and one in ten men over the age of 55 years living in England are known to have troublesome incontinence (Thomas et al 1980). Nearly three-quarters of these are not receiving any help, and yet the amount of money quoted by the Department of Health & Social Security as being spent in hospitals in 1982 on urological disposables such as pads, pants, catheters and urine collecting bags approximated to £60 000 000 per year.

It has been found that among residents of Elderly People's Homes run by the Social Services the prevalence of incontinence is as high as 37% (Bainton et al 1983), and that the number rises rapidly after admission to these homes. The reason for this may be that the incontinence was already a problem but was hidden from the authorities prior to their acceptance to the home because of the social stigma attached to this condition. More likely it is due to the institutionalisation and lack of amenities in strange surroundings which tend to lead to this final degradation. Many of the residents live to be very old and incontinence of urine and faeces together tends to occur at a terminal stage.

Effect of childbearing

Urinary incontinence is known to be far more common among women than among men. From the study undertaken by Thomas et al (1980) it has been shown that incontinence increases with age and with parity. The most dramatic rise is after the first successful pregnancy, and there is then a further upsurge after the fourth child (see Fig. 9.1). Whether this is the result of the pregnancy or parturition has never been satisfactorily proven. Early work by Francis (1960) suggested that symptoms started during pregnancy and continued after childbirth. More recently work by Swash et al (1985) has shown that those women whose babies are delivered by forceps are more likely to have damage to the muscles of the pelvic floor, suggesting that it is at the time of delivery rather than the effect of pregnancy itself that the damage is done. These findings may help to explain the apparent variation in the prevalance of incontinence among women of different races giving birth in many parts of the world.

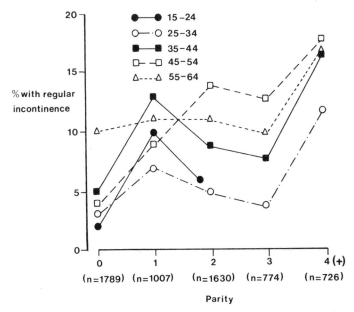

Fig. 9.1 Prevalence in women of regular incontinence (%) — that is, people incontinent twice or more per month — by age and parity. (Reproduced by permission of Dr T. M. Thomas and the British Medical Journal.)

THE ANATOMY AND NORMAL BLADDER FUNCTION

A basic knowledge of the anatomy and normal function of the bladder, urethra and pelvic floor is vital to the understanding of the symptoms which arise in association with dysfunction of the lower urinary tract (Fig. 9.2).

The bladder

The bladder is a hollow organ lying in the pelvis immediately behind the symphysis pubis, and becomes an abdominal structure only when filled. Above, it has the uterus and coils of intestine, posteriorly it is related closely to the cervix and anterior wall of the vagina. Lateral and inferior relations are the structures of the pelvic floor. It receives its arterial supply from branches of the internal iliac arteries, and complex venous plexuses take the blood to the internal iliac veins. There are anastomoses with the ovarian, superior rectal and sacral veins which provide alternative routes to the inferior vena cava.

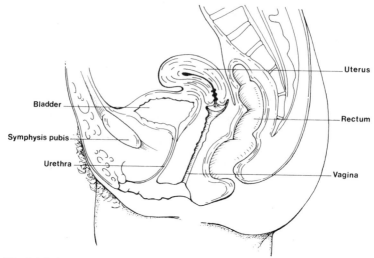

Fig. 9.2 Relations of the female bladder.

Histologically, the wall of the bladder consists of three layers; on the inside is the mucous membrane, on the outer surface the adventitial layer of connective tissue and between them a smooth muscle coat — the detrusor muscle. The mucous membrane consists of an epithelial layer (the urothelium) supported by a coat of loose connective tissue, while the adventitia is composed of bundles of collagen and elastic fibres. Blood vessels, lymphatics and large nerve cells lie among the connective tissue. The detrusor muscle is a meshwork or syncitium of smooth fibres which run in all directions and are without polarity. The interlacing arrangement of these bundles is ideally suited to reduce all dimensions of the bladder lumen upon contraction. In the male the bladder neck should be considered as a separate functional unit. It has been developed as the internal sphincter and has the genital function of preventing retrograde ejaculation of sperms. In the female the muscle fibres of the bladder neck are distinct from those of the detrusor, being of narrow diameter and tightly packed together. They extend obliquely and longitudinally to the urethra (Fig. 9.3).

The urethra

The female urethra extends a distance of 3–4 cm from the bladder neck, lying behind the symphysis pubis and anterior to the vagina.

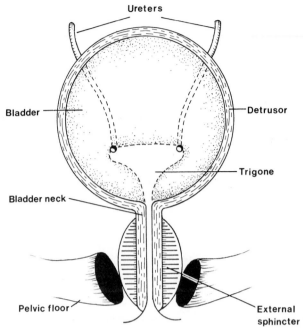

Fig. 9.3. Anatomy of the female bladder.

It passes through the pelvic floor muscles to its orifice on the perineum. The external urethral sphincter — there is no internal sphincter in the female — is anatomically separate from the adjacent peri-urethral striated muscle of the pelvic floor. The fibres form a sleeve which is thickest in the middle of the urethra and are all striated fibres of the slow-twitch variety. This enables the sphincter to maintain a closure pressure on the urethral lumen over prolonged periods without fatigue. It can be considered to be a muscle of posture similar to the soleus muscle in the calf. This function is most important in maintaining continence.

The pelvic floor

The pelvic floor is a diaphragm of muscle and fascia penetrated by the rectum, the urethra and, in the female, the vagina (Fig. 9.4).

It is the pubo-coccygeus of the levator ani muscle which is related to the urethra. Although not an integral part of the urethra, the fibres interdigitate and insert into the lateral walls of the vagina, and by their proximity exert a closing force on the urethral lumen.

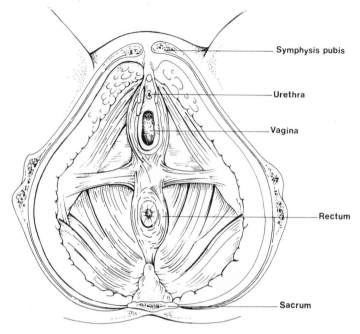

Fig. 9.4 View of female pelvic floor from above showing levator ani muscle.

The muscle fibres are of both the fast- and slow-twitch types. Their contribution to continence is probably important during the sudden increase in abdominal pressure such as coughing and sneezing. They are most effective at a point distal to the maximum urethral closure pressure exerted by the external sphincter.

Pelvic floor function

The function of the pelvic floor is threefold. It prevents eversion of the pelvic viscera, maintains continence of urine and faeces and controls the expulsive activities of the body. In the quadruped, this group of muscles has another subsidiary function — to move the tail. During the course of evolution the animal kingdom has altered its stance from the pronograde to the orthograde position. In order to adapt to the upright posture the contractile properties of the pelvic floor have been exchanged for tensile strength as fascial tissue replaced muscle.

Like any other muscle in the body the pelvic floor or peri-urethral muscles can become fatigued, or damaged, diseased or disused. This can lead to malfunction and atrophy. Similarly this muscle group can be re-educated, hypertrophied and normal function restored or superfunction achieved. Physiologists tell us that the muscles are made up of both slow-twitch and fast-twitch fibres. Both types are capable of adaptation, should their function be altered. Thus it is possible to increase the static postural tone which maintains continence as well as strengthen the rapid response necessary to prevent leakage when a sudden strain is imposed such as a cough or a sneeze.

Neurological control

Neurological control of the bladder should be considered at three different levels — the sacral centre (S.2, 3 & 4) provides the basic reflex arc of micturition with parasympathetic sensory and motor nerves carrying the impulses to and from the bladder. This reflex allows filling and emptying of the bladder, but without co-ordination of the external sphincter. Thus voiding is inefficient and often associated with failure to empty the bladder completely. The second centre is in the pons in the mid-brain and allows co-ordinated and efficient micturition. Lesions between these two centres will lead to dyssynergia such as is found in cases of multiple sclerosis when, despite a normal desire to void and a rise in blader pressure due to the detrusor muscle contracting, the urethral sphincter fails to relax. The third centre, situated in the cerebral cortex, provides the conscious control of voiding. As we mature we learn to inhibit the reflex arc of micturition at will and thus have the ability to void only where and when the social and physical situation is appropriate (Fig. 9.5).

Knowledge of the normal function and neurological control of the bladder leads to a better understanding of the local and systemic lesions which can cause the symptoms associated with the lower urinary tract.

Site of lesions affecting lower urinary tract control:

Brain
Spinal cord
Autonomic nerves
Bladder
Bladder neck
Pelvic floor
Urethra.

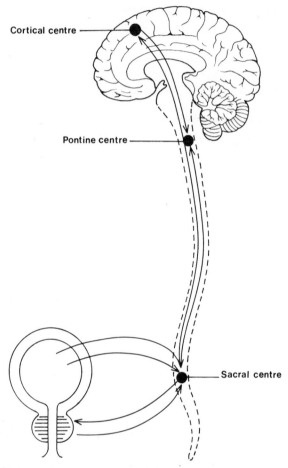

Fig. 9.5 Diagram of nervous control of bladder.

LOWER URINARY TRACT SYMPTOMS

Symptoms associated with lower urinary tract disorders include frequency of micturition, hesitancy of initiation of micturition, disturbances of flow, retention of urine and urinary incontinence. In women, the most common symptom is urinary incontinence. It is a time-honoured tradition that women with urinary dysfunction are referred by their family doctors to the gynaecologist, but that men with a similar condition have created the need for the specialty of urology. Perhaps this is because of the inherent belief that genital prolapse and urinary incontinence go hand in hand. Too often gynaecological notes have consisted of:

c/o Stress incontinence on cough or sneeze.
O.E. Prolapse.
T.C.I. Vaginal hysterectomy & repair.

These two conditions can go together but certainly not in all cases. As an example, it has been noted that among 56 women with significant vaginal prolapse 32% had incontinence due to an incompetent urethral sphincter. Yet of 121 women with incontinence 15% were found to have a significant genital prolapse.

TYPES OF INCONTINENCE

With our improved knowledge of the patho-physiology of the bladder and with the realisation that assessment is of paramount importance we are able to isolate with some accuracy the different types of incontinence. When seeking the cause of incontinence social, psychological and medical factors need to be considered. It is only after careful assessment of the patient and her environment as well as using specific bladder function tests that we can define the cause of incontinence and thus institute effective management.

The Standardisation Committee of the International Continence Society (Bates et al 1976) has defined the symptom of urinary incontinence as being of four main types:

Stress incontinence
Urge incontinence
Reflex incontinence
Overflow incontinence.

Urodynamic studies

The most accurate method of differentiating these types and defining the cause of urinary leakage is by undertaking urodynamic studies. Using transducers to measure pressure it is possible to assess urethral sphincter function and detrusor function while the bladder is filling and emptying.

Stress incontinence

This is most commonly associated with an incompetent urethral sphincter. It is defined as the involuntary loss of urine occurring when the bladder pressure exceeds the maximum urethral pressure in the absence of detrusor activity.

Urge incontinence

This is associated with frequency and urgency of micturition. It occurs when uninhibited detrusor contractions are present either during bladder filling or are provoked by coughing, running or the sound of water. This condition is known as bladder or detrusor instability and is associated with neurological conditions and with bladder outlet obstruction. However, in 30% of women with an unstable bladder the cause is never found (Fig. 9.6).

Reflex incontinence

This is the pathological manifestation of the reflex arc of micturition. It is found, for example, in men and women who are paraplegic. Here, there is a spinal lesion which has severed the cortical control from the local sacral reflex. The bladder empties inefficiently, incompletely and often unconsciously.

Overflow incontinence

As its name suggests, this is associated with an inability to empty

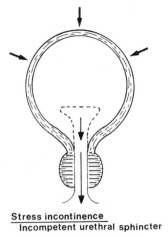

Stress incontinence
Incompetent urethral sphincter

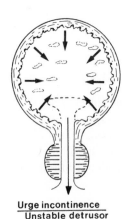

Urge incontinence
Unstable detrusor

Fig. 9.6 Mechanism of stress and urge incontinence.

the bladder completely, leaving a significant volume of residual urine after voiding. This may manifest itself as a constant dribble or as spurts of urine ejected at the time of an extra effort. Usually it is due to bladder outlet or urethral obstruction and is found in men who have prostatic hypertrophy. Obstruction can be found in women due to a retroverted gravid uterus, to pelvic tumours or to urethral stenosis. Overflow incontinence also occurs in men and women who have a large hypotonic floppy bladder which has lost its contractile ability. This can follow radical pelvic surgery, over-distension, or be associated with a diabetic neuropathy.

Urinary incontinence is a symptom. The mechanism of the cause must always be sought. Differentiation into the main groups which are discussed can only be undertaken when urodynamic techniques have been used. Seldom can symptoms be neatly packaged, and many patients have features in common with other groups.

THE AETIOLOGY OF STRESS INCONTINENCE

Stress incontinence is the most common type of leakage found in females. It occurs in 20% of all women seeking help for any type of urinary incontinence. The prevalence among women attending gynaecological clinics throughout the world makes an interesting study. In both Canada (Beck et al 1965) and England (Shepherd 1981) over 30% of women confess to troublesome episodes of stress incontinence, and figures are similar for Australia and New Zealand. Yet among the black people in Zimbabwe and South Africa this type of leakage is rarely seen. Continuous urinary leakage due to vesico-vaginal fistula after obstetric trauma is far more common. In Northern Borneo where the population is mainly of Malay and Chinese origin the prevalence is also very low, and there have been reports from this part of the world that the most common cause is iatrogenic — incontinence occurring after vaginal surgery to repair prolapse.

Urinary incontinence is three times as common in women as it is in men. Why should the male of the species be at such an advantage? Basic anatomy provides one answer. The male pelvic diaphragm is only penetrated by two orifices thus making it a more sound structure. The average functional length of the male urethra is 5 cm, but it is only 3 cm in the female. Pressure studies of the human urethra show that the male has an average resting closure pressure of 80 cm H_2O while the female has an average resting closure pressure of only 50 cm H_2O. Moreover, if a man is asked to contract the muscles of the pelvic floor, not only can he do it without conscious effort but the urethral pressure is doubled. Even a young nulliparous woman is only able to produce an increment of 20% of the resting pressure.

Functional activities provide further information. Small boys are accustomed to competitive games, and discovering the potential of their urinary flow is a constant source of entertainment. They can stop and start their stream without effort. It is only the female pelvis that has to experience the increasing pressure of the enlarging pregnant uterus, the inherent forces of labour and the additional insult and trauma to muscle and fascia involved in episiotomy and instrumental delivery. Only 40% of parous women can stop their flow in mid-stream (Shepherd 1980).

Much has been written on the mental and physiological trauma associated with episiotomy. Very little interest has been taken in the possible effect of episiotomy or lacerations to the perineum on subsequent pelvic floor function. However, recently some work (Snooks et al 1984) discussing the relationship of the pelvic floor to rectal incontinence has suggested that those women who have had a forceps delivery show evidence of muscle fibre denervation. It would seem probable that the pain consequent to any trauma, and particularly that due to stitches in the perineum, may cause immediate protective inhibition of muscle activity. Many women will remember the agony of the first bowel action following a traumatic delivery.

The levator ani muscles of the female have a definite and important function but one which is difficult to isolate and not easy to demonstrate. They only have to be alienated from cortical control for a short while before the brain is unable to renew the pathways voluntarily. With so very little awareness of this muscle group the puerperal woman with a sore perineum rapidly rejects her pelvic floor and the ability to produce an active contraction. The muscles atrophy and are useless.

Why then should there be a geographical difference in the incidence of stress incontinence and how does it relate to pelvic floor function? From South Africa there is a report of a comparative study on urethral and pelvic floor function between three different ethnic races (Knobel 1975). They found that among the black African the bladder neck is placed higher within the abdominal cavity, the functional urethral length is longer and, most interestingly, the muscles of the pelvic floor are capable of greater voluntary effort. Bladder function was found to be less efficient among

Asians and Europeans. As mentioned in the introduction, Kegel (1949) noticed that 30–40% of women were unable to contract their levator ani muscle. Similarly, among English women only 40% have the ability to produce an objective measurement of pressure. Yet it has been found that among a small group of Malay and Chinese 95% of women demonstrated that they had good pelvic floor control (Shepherd 1980).

An explanation of this is not hard to find. The mothers teach their daughters how to use their perineal muscles at the time of puberty — for sexual purposes, but inadvertently perhaps to prevent future incontinence. Another factor which may contribute to this difference in function is their habit of squatting. It is a favourite posture for resting, conversing, eating and micturating. There are few Western women who can admit that this is a comfortable or even possible position to maintain for any length of time. Yet it demands good pelvic floor control to micturate into a hole and it is a natural exercise for the perineal muscles.

Mechanism of stress incontinence

One concept of the cause of stress incontinence is the change in the relationship between the bladder neck and urethra and the pelvic diaphragm (see Fig. 9.7).

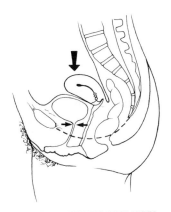
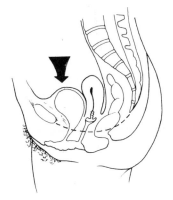

A.   NORMAL POSITION OF BLADDER
     AND PROXIMAL URETHRA

The arrows illustrate the distribution
of pressure on coughing

B.   DESCENT OF BLADDER
     AND PROXIMAL URETHRA

There is no distribution of
pressure on coughing

Fig. 9.7 Mechanism of stress incontinence.

In the normal situation the bladder neck and proximal urethra are above the pelvic floor. In this position any increase in abdominal pressure is equally transmitted to the bladder and to the proximal urethra. The urethral pressure exceeds the bladder pressure both at rest and when the abdominal pressure is increased on effort, such as occurs during coughing or jumping. It is only during the act of voiding that this gradient is reversed. If the bladder and proximal part of the urethra descend below the level of the pelvic diaphragm, as can occur when the ligaments and other structures are stretched during childbirth or lose their elasticity after the menopause, then the closure pressure on the urethra is lost and leakage of urine may result.

PREVENTION OR CURE

Typically it is the multiparous, overweight, menopausal European woman, who is also a smoker with a chronic cough and is taking diuretics, who has frequency of micturition and stress incontinence. Surely we should be looking for ways to prevent this condition from occurring.

Prevention of incontinence

NO EATING
NO SMOKING
NO DRINKING
NO PILLS
NO LAVATORIES

BUT SEX   YES!

Simple measures of prevention include such common sense items as maintenance of an optimum body weight. Additional pressure on a urethral sphincter which is only just competent may be a reversible cause of urinary leakage. Similarly, coughing associated with chronic bronchitis in a habitual cigarette smoker exposes the closure mechanism to an unnecessary degree of repeated strain — so, no smoking. Daily fluid intake needs a balanced outlook. It should be monitored and adjusted to the needs of the individual. Some people who have been advised to drink copiously during an episode of acute urinary tract infection or when catheterised following surgery have continued to have a very high intake (some-times in excess of 10 pints daily). They are distressed by the resulting precipitancy and frequency of voiding, but are reluctant to ignore the orders of the doctor which have never been countermanded.

Certain fluids such as tea, coffee, orange or tomato juice are irritant to some bladders and individual sensitivities must be researched. In contrast, some people, elderly women in particular, feel that they should reduce their fluids for fear of an embarrassing accident. Concentrated urine has an irritant effect on the bladder which responds by an early desire to empty. Adequate fluids are necessary, and an intake equivalent to 6 to 8 cups daily should be recommended.

Injudicious pharmacology may be a cause of bladder symptoms. It has been estimated that at least 50% of men and women over the age of 70 years are being prescribed diuretics to treat either hypertension or pendent oedema. Diuretics are designed to reduce body fluids and result in increased renal and bladder function. Frequency of voiding is increased and is often associated with extreme precipitancy. Unaccustomed urgency of micturition in the elderly whose mobility or dexterity may be impaired can result in embarrassing incontinence. Imagine having had a stroke and preparing yourself to void in a hurry when you cannot use half your body!

Another group of drugs affecting bladder control are the sedatives. Given unwittingly to a patient who is accustomed to voiding regularly during the night, the depth of sleep may cause them not to wake when the normal desire to void occurs. This can result in leakage on the way to the lavatory or even to a wet bed. These are examples of some of the unwanted effects of drugs which are not always considered or explained when prescribed.

Why should a style of lavatory be a possible preventable cause of urinary incontinence among women living in the Western world? Experience has led to an impression that stress incontinence is rare among black Africans and among Malay and Chinese people living in their own countries. Reasons are difficult to find but certainly lavatory seats are a rarity among native people and they squat to void. To undertake this it is necessary to have control of the urinary stream. If aim is poor and the receptacle is missed, the ability to stop and start the stream is required. Pelvic floor muscles are used in this manoeuvre and are known to be much more effective and under better voluntary control than among most Europeans. The design of a lower lavatory bowl putting the user into a nearer approximation to the squatting position would be an improvement on the traditional model. A similar effect can be had by putting the feet up on a stool while sitting on the lavatory seat.

MANAGEMENT

Surgery, drug therapy and bladder training as well as re-education of the pelvic floor muscles are all included in the armamentarium of treatment of urinary incontinence. For some sufferers appliances, pads and pants and catheters will be necessary. These should be used as an adjunct to regaining continence or, failing that, to provide social acceptance.

Having made full social, psychological and medical assessment of the cause of bladder dysfunction an initial plan of treatment can be made (see Fig. 9.8).

SURGERY

The choice of patient

When selecting patients for surgery the important points to remember are their quality of life rather than their age, their plans for future childbearing, whether they are overweight and if they have chronic respiratory tract disease. The majority of women referred for surgery are between 45 and 55 years. However, it is the older members of our society who have the greatest problem, and provided the patient is co-operative and fit for anaesthetic, age is no contra-indication to surgery.

If the patient plans to have more babies, then almost certainly the operation should be deferred since it is the first surgical procedure which has the highest success rate. Should surgery be necessary and post-operative urinary control is good, Caesarian section may have to be considered as the subsequent method of delivery.

Previous mention has been made of the hazard of obesity and how incontinence can be cured by weight loss. Gross obesity makes surgery technically difficult as well as increasing the risk of anaesthetic and post-operative problems. Similarly, to undertake surgery on a patient who has a cough is asking for a stormy post-operative course and a poor result.

Choice of operation

Over a hundred operations have been described — all designed to

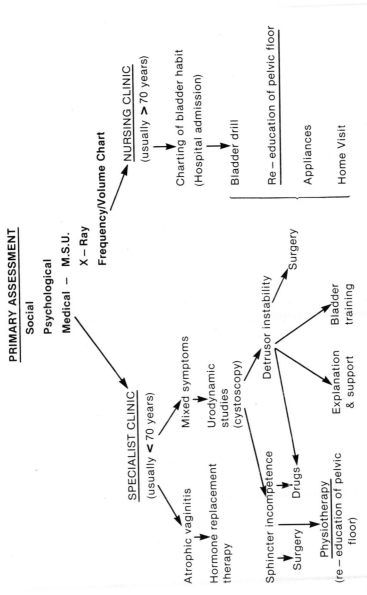

Fig. 9.8 Suggested management for female patients with urinary incontinence.

cure urinary incontinence. This is an indication of our lack of understanding of the mechanism involved and also of the disenchantment of both surgeon and patient with the results of surgery.

The two best-known methods involve either a suprapubic incision for a colposuspension or a vaginal approach in the case of an anterior repair. Personal experience often determines the method which the surgeon selects. If there is a symptomatic prolapse of the uterus, bladder or rectum this will need to be corrected at the time of the operation. Hysterectomy may need to be performed for gynaecological reasons and, depending on the size and mobility of the uterus, either an abdominal or a vaginal approach will be used.

There are many modifications of these two techniques, some favoured by urologists and some by gynaecologists. Most women will benefit from a surgical approach for the management of their stress incontinence, but it must be remembered that there are conservative methods which can be usefully employed. If surgery is the method of choice, it has been found that the cure rate is greatly enhanced by pre- and post-operative pelvic floor re-education.

DRUG THERAPY

Drug therapy in the management of urinary incontinence is usually restricted to those patients who complain of urge incontinence and have been found to have an 'unstable bladder' due to uninhibited contraction of the detrusor muscle. The unstable bladder presents a difficult therapeutic problem. This is clear from the variety of measures that have been tried. Many drugs with differing actions have been recommended. The main types include the anticholinergics such as propantheline and emepronium bromide — both with significant side-effects and great variation in their absorption. Musculotrophic drugs such as flavoxate and imipramine may be helpful. Others have been used but the optimum medical treatment with maximum specific action and minimal side-effects has yet to be found.

BLADDER TRAINING

Frewen (1980) and Jarvis (1982) have written of the use of bladder drill for those women with ideopathic detrusor instability. They claim symptomatic and objective improvement in 80% of patients.

Other retraining techniques include biofeedback, hypnosis, acupuncture and psychotherapy.

PELVIC FLOOR RE-EDUCATION

When urinary incontinence is due to pelvic floor dysfunction or urethral sphincter incompetence, re-educating the peri-urethral muscles (levator ani) has an important part to play in management. Treatment can consist of electrical stimulation alone, exercise alone or a combination of both techniques.

Electrical treatment

The rationale behind electrical stimulation as a method of treatment is that it increases the blood supply, may break down fine adhesions following surgery, increases the resting urethral tone of the muscles and, most importantly, restores cortical awareness. Thus, the patient is able to relate to her pelvic floor and this will assist her in regaining voluntary control.

Previously, the current used to stimulate the muscle fibres of the levator ani was faradism. In some centres interferential therapy has become popular. This is an alternating current of medium frequency and low intensity. By using two currents of differing frequency so that their paths cross as they pass through the body a combined effect is produced. It is this modified current which stimulates motor nerves and muscle fibres. As yet, no controlled study using this technique has proved its usefulness. Most therapists involved in muscle re-education still use the interrupted direct current where it is possible to vary the current in intensity, pulse duration and pulse rate. It has been shown that the use of an internal electrode is the most effective way to stimulate the pubo-coccygeus, and yet there are at least five different ways of applying the electrodes externally, all of which are in common use (Scott et al 1969).

Some trials have been conducted using electrical stimulation alone. Brown (1980) compared different forms of physiotherapy using an objective assessment and found that electrical stimulation was of no particular value. His results agreed with those of Wilson et al (1984) who presented his results on the value of physiotherapy in the treatment of stress incontinence. He stated that the addition of interferential therapy and faradism did not appear to confer significant benefit over pelvic floor exercises alone.

Exercise

To use the word exercise in the re-education of the pelvic floor is to be misleading. To prevent leakage of urine the muscles of the pelvic floor must be in a constant state of awareness and must be able to respond quickly to a sudden increase in abdominal pressure. A scheme of graded exercises such as are given for restoration of function in any muscle group (e.g. quadriceps after meniscectomy) is essential but useless if not associated with a clear understanding and a persisting motivation from the patient. Studies (Shepherd 1981) have shown a success rate in excess of 80% on long term follow-up of patients who have been assessed properly and taught correctly.

An interesting presentation by Klarskow et al (1984) compared surgery with physiotherapy in a controlled trial. They showed that only 42% of patients were satisfied following a retraining programme and concluded that surgery was superior to pelvic floor re-education. This low success rate is perhaps explained by lack of specificity in their selection of cases and the absence of objective assessment during the exercise programme which in itself was inadequate. However, they emphasised the most important fact that the majority of patients will benefit from this method of treatment and that surgery may be avoided in about one third of cases.

Perhaps the best management is to combine these two methods of electrical stimulation and muscle re-education. Ideally, all treatment should be given on a one-to-one basis, although after the initial visit it may be possible to conduct these exercises in small groups. The first attendance will occupy the longest time since the success depends greatly on the patient's understanding and motivation. Full explanation of the mechanism of continence together with the plans for the course of treatment are required. Following this, a few minutes using a vaginal electrode with interrupted direct current will provide tactile sensation and renew cortical awareness of the pelvic floor contraction. This will lead to a scheme of graded exercises, varying in the number, duration and intensity of each contraction.

Before and during treatment the function of the muscles needs assessment. Using urodynamic techniques, this can be done by measuring urethral pressure during the resting phase and during contraction. More simply, this can be done with great accuracy and repeatability using digital assessment. Either the patient or the therapist should insert two fingers into the vagina in order to feel

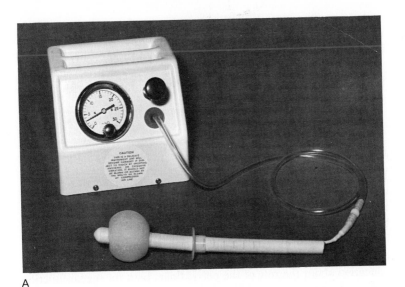

A

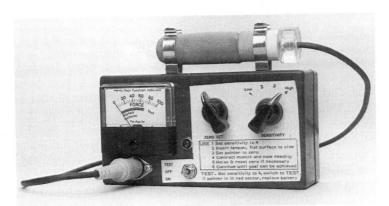

B

Fig. 9.9 Illustrations of prototype perineometers or vaginal exercisers.

the vaginal wall tightening during voluntary contraction. This is the only way to prevent trick movements which are legion when the particular muscle group is under surveillance.

Muscle strength may also be tested by a perineometer (Fig. 9.9). Various pieces of equipment, all variations of that originally produced by Kegel (1948), have been designed. Few are available and the perfect measuring device has yet to be manufactured. As an adjunct to exercises the perineometer can be used to assess progress, and patients appreciate the added motivation (Shepherd et al 1983, Castleden et al 1983). Successful results depend on correct selection of patients who are well motivated, together with enlightened teaching.

FURTHER EDUCATION

For the majority, incontinence should be considered as a preventable disorder. Certainly there are many factors that predispose to the condition which, when it strikes, is not only a personal disaster but one which affects relatives, carers and the entire community. This is the age of positive health and preventative medicine. Early enlightenment for our future mothers must be the answer. Perhaps education about the role of the pelvic floor, both for sexual function and in the maintenance of continence, should be stressed to our teenagers. It could be included with other sex education. Those promoting health, supervising yoga classes and the more energetic aerobic exercises must give thought to this muscle group. Well Women's clinics are becoming a necessity for every forward-looking community and yet no importance is given to preventing incontinence by simple advice and teaching. A woman should be constantly aware of her pelvic floor and of its purpose. Only then will these muscles not become alienated and useless at the first insult such as a traumatic birth or a septic episiotomy.

We are fortunate in having three groups of professonals who have done much to improve the understanding of bladder dysfunction and of urinary incontinence in particular. The Association of Chartered Physiotherapists in Obstetrics and Gynaecology was formed as a specialist group. Annual meetings together with recognised courses have resulted in many physiotherapists being enthusiastic protagonists of pelvic floor re-education. The International Continence Society has met annually for the past 16 years and aims to encourage research and provide a forum for a wide exchange of ideas. More recently, a multi-disciplinary group of nurses, physiotherapists, doctors and others have formed the Association of Continence Advisors. With the support of these three bodies there is renewed enthusiasm among the professional carers. The technical advances in prevention, assessment and management make urinary incontinence a condition which should not occur, but if it does it may be cured and certainly can be contained. What we require is a better informed society and more caring professionals.

REFERENCES

Bainton D, Edgington A, Shepherd A M 1983 'D' is for Dignity. Health & Social Service Journal Jan. 50–51

Bates P, Bradley W E 1976 International Continence Society — First Report on the standardisation of terminology of lower urinary tract function. British Journal of Urology 48: 39–41

Beck R P, Hsu N 1965 Pregnancy, childbirth and the menopause related to the development of stress incontinence. Journal of Obstetrics & Gynaecology 91: 820–822

Brown A D G 1980 Physiotherapy. Communication to the Annual Meeting of the International Uro-gynaecological Association. New Orleans

Castleden G M, Duffin H M, Mitchell E P 1984 The effect of physiotherapy on stress incontinence. Age & Aging 13: 235–237

Francis W J 1960 Disturbances of bladder function in relation to pregnancy. Journal of Obstetrics & Gynaecology British Empire 67: 353–366

Frewen W K 1980 Management of urgency and frequency of micturition. British Journal of Urology 52: 367–369

Green-Armytage V B 1948 The role of physiotherapy in Obstetrics & Gynaecology. Journal of Obstetrics & Gynaecology British Empire 52: 21–23

Jarvis G J 1982 The management of urinary incontinence due to primary vesical sensory urgency by bladder drill. British Journal of Urology 54: 374–376

Kegel A H 1948 Progressive resistance exercise in functional restoration of the perineal muscles. American Journal of Obstetrics & Gynaecology 56: 238–248

Kegel A H 1949 The physiologic treatment of poor tone and function of genital muscles and of urinary stress incontinence. Western Journal of Surgery 57: 527–535

Klarskow P, Belving D, Bischoff N, Dorph S, Gerstengerg T, Hald T, Hjortkjaer P, Okholm B, Tikjob G, Wormslev M 1984 Pelvic floor exercises versus surgery for female urinary stress incontinence. Preliminary report. Proceedings of International Continence Society XIV Meeting, Innsbruck, 159–161

Knobel J 1975 Stress incontinence in the black female. South African Medical Journal 49: 430–432

Scott B O, Green J, Couldrey B M 1969 Pelvic faradism. Investigation of methods. Physiotherapy 55: 302–305

Shepherd A M 1980 In: Mandelstam D (ed) Incontinence and its management. Croom Helm, Kent, pp 156–159

Shepherd A M 1981 Other aspects of urinary incontinence. In: Jordan J A, Stanton S L (ed) The incontinent woman. Royal College of Gynaecologists, London, pp 89–92

Shepherd A M, Montgomery E, Anderson R S 1983 A pilot study of a pelvic exerciser in women with stress incontinence. Journal of Obstetrics & Gynaecology 3: 201–202

Snooks S J, Setchell M, Swash M, Henry M M 1984 Injury to innervation of pelvic floor sphincter musculature in childbirth. The Lancet Sept 8: 546–550

Swash M, Snooks S J, Henry M M 1985 Unifying concept of pelvic floor disorders and incontinence. Journal of the Royal Society of Medicine 78: 906–911

Thomas T M, Plymat K E, Blannin J, Meade T W 1980 Prevalence of urinary incontinence. British Medical Journal 281: 1243–1245

Wilson P D, Al Samarral T, Deakin M, Kolbe E, Brown A D G 1984 The value of physiotherapy in female genuine stress incontinence. Proceedings, International Continence Society XIV Meeting, Innsbruck, pp 156–157

Annotated bibliography

For the convenience of the user this bibliography has been divided into obstetrics and gynaecology after an initial short list of texts common to both. Since, however, the subjects are interlinked, the division is bound to be somewhat arbitrary. Both sections include textbooks by therapists and medical specialists. A selection of original papers (to some of which reference has been made by contributors) is also listed.

Obstetric practice is an ever-changing branch of medicine, and the physiotherapist depends largely on papers in medical journals and reports of conferences to keep abreast with current thought. In gynaecology the newest developments are in the field of incontinence. Its management is multi-disciplinary with physiotherapists, nurses and medical specialists becoming increasingly involved. Literature is sparse owing to the fact that studies are comparatively recent. The proceedings of the annual meeting of the International Continence Society are published each year, providing a useful source of up-to-date information.

The listing of a book or paper in this bibliography does not necessarily mean that the editor endorses its conclusions. Some controversial items are included in order to stimulate reflection and discussion.

TEXTS RELATED TO OBSTETRICS AND GYNAECOLOGY

CIBA collection of medical illustrations 1954 Volume 2 Reproductive system. CIBA, New Jersey.
 The atlas consists of drawings by Frank Netter — an excellent medical artist — and a text compiled from several medical disciplines. It is of value for anyone interested in obstetrics and gynaecology, but the section on the pelvic floor is particularly useful. The drawings are explicit and enable the reader to visualise this complicated area of muscles and surrounding structures.

Collins M G (ed) 1987 Women's health through lifestages — a physiotherapist's role and contribution. Australian Physiotherapy Association (NSW Branch).

The publication of this book, with chapters by various physiotherapists practising in Australia, has been designed to coincide with the 1987 World Congress of Physical Therapy in Sydney. It surveys the help the physiotherapist can give to a woman through the phases of her life. The introduction discusses aspects of general health; subsequent chapters trace a course through childbirth to the post-menopausal period and the various problems which may arise. A list of objectives at the head of each chapter makes an easy reference device for the reader. There is much practical information and a positive approach underlining the preventive aspect of physiotherapy in obstetrics and gynaecology. It is doubtful whether any benefit is to be gained by patients' descriptions of their cases and the inclusion of so many weakens the book. However, this ambitious project is sufficiently successful to make it worth including in a volume which surveys the international scene.

England M A 1983 A colour atlas of life before birth. Wolfe Medical Publications, London.

There can surely be no finer illustrations of the course of fetal development in utero than these photographs, all taken from human specimens and dissections. After a series showing the growth of the fetus up to term with photographs of ultrasound scans from week 12 to week 33, the author traces the development of the individual organs and parts. Labelling is clear and each section starts with a brief written introduction. The book ends with a short chapter on childbirth with photographs of the pelvis and skull illustrating the movements of the head during normal delivery.

Llewellyn-Jones D 1986 Fundamentals of obstetrics and gynaecology (2 vols), 4th edn. Faber and Faber, London.

This double volume by the Associate Professor in Obstetrics and Gynaecology at Sydney University was first published in 1969 and has remained the authoritative textbook for students. The fourth edition has new sections including antenatal screening, perinatal bereavement and the examination of the neonate, and re-written sections on premenstrual and perimenstrual syndromes as well as revisions in most chapters.

It is a pity that the short section on childbirth education has not been up-dated in line with current practice. That apart, the physiotherapist specializing in the subjects will find this an ideal book to have beside her.

Philipp E E, Barnes J, Newton M (eds) 1986 Scientific foundations of obstetrics and gynaecology. Heinemann, London.

This book can be highly recommended to anyone seeking the most up-to-date information on obstetrics and gynaecology. First published in 1970, it was re-issued with revisions in 1977 and 1986. The editors (two from the United Kingdom and one from the United States) have produced a truly international volume by drawing their contributors from many different countries, all of whom are authorities on the latest advances in their subjects. Physiotherapists will particularly appreciate the account of the structure and function of the pelvic floor (authors from Australia and South Africa) and the chapter on Maternal Positions in Labour (authors from Chicago). An absorbing new chapter written by the editors on the Ethical and Legal Aspects of Medical Research includes a discussion on the problems posed by in vitro fertilization and the use of fetal material in research. A useful glossary of scientific terms and abbreviations has also been added to this latest edition.

GYNAECOLOGY

Gosling J S, Dixon J R, Humpherson J A (eds) 1983 Functional anatomy of the urinary tract, an integrated text and colour atlas. Churchill Livingstone, Edinburgh, New York.

The section on the lower urinary tract, including the gross and microscopic anatomy of the urethra, is of particular interest. The text is detailed and includes the latest research on the lower urinary tract. The illustrations are colourful and clear. The anatomists have worked closely with clinical specialists who have provided the human material. Each illustration is accompanied by explanatory labelled diagrams.

Henry M M, Swash M (eds) 1985 Coloproctology and the pelvic floor. Pathophysiology and management. Butterworths, London.

This book edited by a rectal surgeon and neurologist, while mainly for a medical readership, is of great interest to therapists concerned with the pelvic floor. The editors have researched in this field using new techniques. They bring together a body of information from a number of contributors on the anatomy and physiology of the levator ani and the external and internal sphincters, with special consideration being given to the mechanism of continence and defaecation. Other chapters include methods of investigation, pelvic floor disorders and their management and faecal incontinence.

International Continence Society, c/o Urology, Southmead Hospital, Bristol, UK.

The proceedings of the annual meetings are published each year. The scientific sessions include papers from urologists, gynaecologists, geriatricians, nurses and others. The main impetus to these sessions has been the development of urodynamic investigations enabling objective studies of bladder function to be performed.

Jordan J A, Stanton S L (eds) 1981 The incontinent woman. Proceedings of a scientific meeting of the Royal College of Obstetricians and Gynaecologists.

The papers on the management of incontinence are multidisciplinary and reflect areas of clinical importance and development. Contributions are from urologist, gynaecologist, neurologist and geriatrician. The paper on the Treatment of Stress Incontinence by Physiotherapy was followed by discussion in which several obstetric physiotherapists participated. The discussion is recorded.

Mandelstam D (ed) 1986 Incontinence and its management, 2nd edn. Croom Helm, London.

This book, edited by a therapist continence adviser and first produced in 1980, has become a standard work for a broad-based multidisciplinary perspective on incontinence. Contributors include medical and nursing personnel, a social worker, clinical psychologist and therapist. The second edition (1986) brings the nursing section up-to-date on an aspect of care which is rapidly developing. There is also a chapter on the prevalence and health service implications of incontinence.

Norton C 1986 Nursing for continence. Beaconsfield Publishers Ltd, Bucks, UK.

This is the first book of its kind written for nurses and other health professionals. The author focuses on individual patient care using research evidence whenever it is available. The particular requirements of different patients are dealt with in separate chapters on children, women, men, the elderly, the disabled and the mentally handicapped. Detailed advice is given on practical aspects of care, with descriptions of the therapeutic tools which can be used to promote continence.

Journal of the Chartered Society of Physiotherapy 1983 (supplement) Incontinence.

This supplement includes a number of articles published in the Journal. There are several by therapists on the treatment of stress incontinence, two medical contributions on bladder dysfunction, investigation, and management of incontinence, and one by a nurse on the role of the continence adviser. The more general role of the therapist is also considered in relation to incontinence, and a select bibliography is included.

Stanton S L (ed) 1984 Clinical gynaecologic urology. C V Mosby Company, St Louis, USA.

In the UK gynaecological urology is now a sub-speciality of obstetrics and gynaecology. Stuart Stanton, a gynaecologist with a long standing interest in the subject of incontinence, brings together experts not only in gynaecology and urology but also many others with a common interest in the subject. Chapters include those on anatomy, neurophysiology, pharmacology, urodynamic investigations, bladder malfunction, the elderly, psychiatric aspects, as well as specialist nursing and therapy contributions.

OBSTETRICS

Arns C 1986 Low back pain in labour — a trial using TENS. Australian Physiotherapy Association's Journal of the National Group in Obstetrics & Gynaecology 5 (2): October 1986.

A clinical trial of TENS was carried out on 18 labouring women who complained of low back pain early in labour. This was compared with 10 randomly selected who had the backache but no TENS. Dual channel TENS units were used and assessment of their use was made as soon as possible after delivery, usually within 12 hours. Pain relief was categorised as slight, moderate or marked. All women who used the TENS felt some relief of low back pain, with 11 out of 18 gaining marked relief and 7 moderate relief. Of the 14 who required another adjunctive analgesic, it was most usually for anterior or suprapubic pain. A willingness to use TENS in subsequent labours was expressed by all women.

Brice Pitt D 1978 Enjoying motherhood. Sheldon Press, London.

The author (a doctor and a father) traces the changing emotions of a woman through the three trimesters of her pregnancy and the period of her homecoming with the new baby. Starting with her reaction to discovering she is pregnant (which may be ambivalent) he discusses her anxieties, relating them to the changes taking place in her body, the baby, the birth and the hospital. Mixed feelings and worries about the whole event are more common than many couples realise and they need to be forewarned. Emotional reassurance is an essential component of an antenatal preparation programme, and anyone involved in this work will find this book an invaluable guide to this most important aspect of parenthood education.

Dobzhansky T, Ayala F J, Stebbins G L, Valentine J 1977 Evolution. W H Freeman, San Francisco.

This book is an up-to-date resumé of anthropologists' findings that tell the story of human evolution. The authors delve into factors which have tended to make childbirth difficult, and explore the tantalising supposition that Neanderthal man may have succumbed to an impossible birth situation. Paedomorphism, the persistance of some infantile characteristics into adulthood, is put forward as one of the success factors in the emergence of mankind.

DonTigny R L 1985 Function and pathomechanics of the sacro-iliac joint. A review. Physical Therapy 65 (1)

In this excellent article the author describes his understanding of the biomechanics and function of the sacro-iliac joint and the dysfunction and pathomechanics of the joint as a common cause of low back pain. He discusses a simple assessment procedure, associated pain mechanisms, treatment and prevention of the problem, and related literature. Anterior and posterior rotation of the innominate on the sacrum is particularly clearly described. The paper is helpfully illustrated and well referenced.

Flynn A M, Kelly J, Hollins G, Lynch P F 1978 Ambulation in labour. British Medical Journal 2: 591–593

This is a report of a randomised study undertaken at the Birmingham Maternity Hospital of 68 women in spontaneous labour, half of whom were ambulant and half recumbant during the first stage of labour. The second and third stages were managed in bed for both groups. The results showed that in the ambulant group contractions were less frequent but stronger, the first stage significantly shorter and the need for augmentation and analgesia less. In addition there were more normal deliveries in the ambulant group and the Apgar scores were higher. The conclusion was that ambulance should be encouraged and mention was made of the interesting fact that this was recommended by William Smellie as long ago as 1748.

Gillet J 1979 Childbirth in Pithiviers, France. Lancet, October 27th

This is an account by a midwife of a visit to Dr Michel Odent's Maternity Unit where she witnessed eight births. Today in the United Kingdom the demand for a return to home births is heard from time to time as a reaction against the clinical situation in the hospital. In this unit it would seem that a compromise has been achieved by the creation of a homely atmosphere (curtains at the windows of the labour room, a record player available and medical equipment well out of sight). Maximum freedom is permitted to the woman and her partner, and a high degree of personal care is given by attendants already well known to the pair. The use of drugs and medical intervention are reported to be minimal and favourable statistics quoted for the years 1977 and 1978. Happily, some aspects of the care described, such as ambulance in early labour and choice of delivery positions, operate in many units today.

Grieve G P 1976 The sacro-iliac joint. Physiotherapy 62 (12)

Although published 10 years ago, the masterly coverage of all aspects of the joint and its care must make this paper one of the most useful and used papers ever written; it is also one of very few that dares to address backache in pregnancy. All obstetric physiotherapists should have read and marked it. Anatomy and anomalies, movement and posture, trauma and disease, assessment and treatment are thoroughly explored, discussed and referenced.

Grieve G P 1981 Common vertebral joint problems. Churchill Livingstone, Edinburgh.

This is the bible for any physiotherapist attempting to understand and treat back pain or malfunction. Anatomy, physiology, assessment, treatment and much else is addressed fully and with much wisdom. Every physiotherapy school and department of any size should own a copy. With 1400 references from all the respected sources it is an unparalleled 'source book' for those researching into any aspect of vertebral problems.

Haddad F 1982 Alternative positions for labour. Midwife, Health Visitor & Community Nurse 18: 290–4.

This article is by an obstetrician who encourages women to remain ambulant in early labour and adopt upright postures of their choice for delivery. She gives a brief history of the changes in birthing positions which have occurred at different times and in different societies. She describes the proven benefits of the new approach to positioning, citing international authorities, and gives details of the management of labour conducted according to these theories. This account is highly recommended to the obstetric physiotherapist, not least for the extensive reference list which forms a useful guide to the relevant literature on the subject.

Harrison R F, Woods T, Shore M, Mathews G, Unwin A 1986 Pain relief in labour using transcutaneous electrical nerve stimulation (TENS). British Journal of Obstetrics & Gynaecology 93: 739–746.

A double blind controlled trial using TENS and TENS placebo was undertaken at the Rotunda Hospital, Dublin. 100 primigravidae and 50 women experiencing their third labour took part. Pain levels were assessed during labour at hourly intervals and comments taken from the mothers one hour and twenty-four hours after delivery. The conclusion reached was that pain assessed during labour and the need for additional analgesia showed no significant difference between the two groups. However, consumer satisfaction as revealed by the post-labour questioning was significantly greater in the TENS group. The authors concluded that there is a place for TENS as pain relief in labour but suggested the need for an improved design of machine which might have greater effects on the intense level of labour pain.

Kitzinger S 1984 The experience of childbirth. Penguin Books, London.

Sheila Kitzinger (an anthropologist and mother of five) is on the advisory panel of the National Childbirth Trust and has a world reputation as teacher, lecturer and writer. This, her most famous book, was first published in 1962 and has been in print (with revisions) since then. In it she emphasises the importance of the harmony between the bodily functions and the emotions and the psycho-sexual aspect of childbirth. She has been influential in the changing attitudes towards women and birth and her book should be read by all childbirth educators, notwithstanding some of the controversial issues presented.

Kropej H 1984 Fundamentals of ear acupuncture, 2nd edn. Karl F Hang Verlag GmbH and Company, Heidelberg.

This is a highly recommended book for reading and reference on the latest developments in auriculotherapy. It contains clear diagrams of ear acupuncture points with their location and uses, without specifying the points to use in particular conditions.

Leboyer F 1975 Birth without violence. Fontana/Collins, UK.

This is a translation of a book first published in France by Leboyer who was until recently chef du clinique in the Paris Faculty of Medicine. The author considers the influence on the newborn of the environment of the birth. He describes the possible effects of bright lights, noise and brisk handling in the delivery room. He talks of the 'tragic' expression, tight-shut eyes and twitching limbs of the howling baby and questions whether this is acceptable. His recommendations are a semi-darkened room, peace, the baby delivered onto the mother's stomach and the umbilical cord left intact until pulsation has ceased. The book has photographs of babies (many by the author) which vividly illustrate his theories. The increasingly peaceful atmosphere in today's labour wards and gentle handling of the baby is in part due to the pioneer work of Leboyer.

MacLennan A M 1981 Relaxin. A review. Australian and New Zealand Journal of Obstetrics & Gynaecology 21 (4).

This recent review helpfully elucidates relaxin and its actions for the non-endocrinologist. It traces the historical development of knowledge of the substance and presents the research evidence. The paper was acknowledged by Professor F Greenwood and his wife — both internationally known and much respected researchers in this field.

Maitland G D 1986 Vertebral manipulation, 5th edn. Butterworths, London.
This new substantially re-written edition of the standard text would be an invaluable learning and revisionary resource for the obstetric physiotherapist to increase her knowledge and skills prior to using these oscillatory techniques in the treatment of carefully selected cases of backache in pregnancy. As Professor D A Brewerton contends in Chapter 2, 'It is true that pregnancy presents mechanical and technical problems, but if marked pain is clearly originating within the spine, there is no absolute bar to manipulation provided sensible precautions are taken'.

Mitchell L 1985 Simple relaxation. John Murray, London.
This book, which has been in print since 1977, introduces the method of relaxation most commonly practised in obstetric units in the United Kingdom and many other countries of the world. The author describes the typical pattern of tension and explains the physiological basis of her method for releasing this. The reader will learn from the book how to apply the technique of relaxation to him/herself before teaching it to others. Mitchell suggests how her method can be applied to various conditions and situations. One of these is the childbearing period encompassing pregnancy, labour and the puerperium. Since its physiological basis makes it independent of surroundings, this type of relaxation has been found by many to surpass all others in the busy labour ward situation.

Noble E 1982 Essential exercises for the childbearing year. Houghton Mifflin, Boston; John Murray, London.
The author founded the Obstetric and Gynaecology Section of the American Physical Therapy Association and has an international reputation as writer and lecturer. She has always advocated special exercise programmes for the antenatal as well as the postnatal period. In this book, which includes a chapter on Caesarian birth, she describes techniques of exercise, breathing and relaxation related to pregnancy, labour and the puerperium. She gives a lucid account of the anatomical structures relevant to childbearing and the changes occurring in them. She describes movements which may be performed and those which must be avoided — all illustrated with clear, attractive figures. Throughout she emphasises the very positive effects of physical fitness in minimising the stresses of childbearing. A useful illustrated summary of all the exercises is given at the end of this comprehensive and readable book, which is invaluable for the childbirth educator.

Nogier P M F 1969 Treatise de auriculo-therapie. Maisonneuve, Moulins-les-Metz, France.
An interesting and easy to read book which plots the course and development of auricular acupuncture as practised by Nogier. Treatments are amply illustrated by actual case studies. Advice is given on the practical aspects of the subject including examination and the interpretation and recording of observations.

O'Driscoll 1975 An obstetrician's view of pain. British Journal of Anaesthesia 47: 1053.
This is an exposition of the 'Active Management of Labour' as practised at the National Maternity Hospital, Dublin. When a woman is admitted to this hospital she is promised the continuous support of her own nurse and that she

will deliver within eight hours of the start of her labour. If progress is too slow this will involve artificial rupture of the membranes and acceleration with oxytocin infusion. Professor O'Driscoll shows a sympathetic awareness of the emotional needs of the labouring woman and relates the need for pain relief to lack of personal support and length of labour. Despite the laudability of his views, many women wishing to have some control over the course of their labour will find such intervention as may be necessary unacceptable and the issue remains a controversial one.

Russell J G B 1982 The rationale of primitive delivery positions. British Journal of Obstetrics & Gynaecology 89: 712–715.

Women are increasingly being encouraged to deliver in one of the upright positions (although as Noble mentions there are still units where the supine habit persists). The work of Russell has been highly influential in the change in policy. In this paper he suggests that one third of women in the world give birth with no medical help available and that such women find for themselves the most advantageous position viz. upright. He gives the radiological evidence of the increase in the pelvic outlet (28%) in the squatting as opposed to the supine posture, and traces the history of methods of delivery from the earliest records. Illustrations are dramatic and all show the woman using one of the upright postures. This paper should be studied by all childbirth educators who need to adapt their labour preparation to train the expectant mother for what may be unfamiliar postures.

Steer C M 1975 Moloy's evaluation of the pelvis in obstetrics. Plenum Medical Book Company, New York.

This book represents many years of research into male and female pelvic differences, female pelvic types, the relationship between fetal head and maternal pelvis and the likelihood of serious arrest in both classic and mixed types of pelvis. Although ultrasound scanning is now providing more data on feto-pelvic proportions, the usefulness of this comprehensive book on pelvic anatomy cannot be over-estimated.

Voll R 1976 Electro-acupuncture. 5 vols. Medizinisch Literarische Verlag GmbH, West Germany.

Five volumes of work for the advanced student of electro-acupuncture, giving very detailed information on the scientific development and evidence to support the use of acupuncture and electrotherapy. The author gives a full account of electro-physiology, neuro-physiology and neuro-therapy. The treatment approach is very objective. The replacement of needles by electrotherapy is discussed and the greater acceptability this has both to patient and practitioner.

Whiteford B, Polden M 1984 Postnatal exercises. Century, London.

Two physiotherapists with special experience in obstetrics give a programme of exercises for the new mother during the first six months after delivery. The physical and emotional state of the new mother is realistically described in the opening chapters. The importance of correct posture in relation to back care is pointed out, and the place of relaxation in the new mother's busy life explained. A progressive series of exercises follows, with step-by-step instructions: many of these exercises can be done with the baby, as is demonstrated by a number of beautiful photographs. Besides exercises, there is a wealth of wide-ranging practical advice: on lifting, carrying, nursing the baby, for example, and (for the post-Caesarean mother) on getting in and out of bed.

The book is primarily designed for new mothers, who will find the simple anatomical diagrams and illustrations easy to follow. But it is also highly recommended for physiotherapists, who will find in it all the help they need in teaching the new mothers under their care.

Williams M, Booth D 1985 Antenatal education — guidelines for teachers, 3rd edn. Churchill Livingstone, London.
   Written by an obstetric physiotherapist and a midwife, and first published in 1974, this is the definitive textbook and reference book for the antenatal teacher. It contains a wealth of practical information relating to teaching techniques, and instruction on the planning and equipping of classes and the use of visual aids. All aspects of pregnancy are discussed and antenatal tests explained. After a description of labour (both normal and complicated) there is a chapter on the puerperium and babycare. In every instance the authors give a full account aimed at the antenatal teacher and also, most importantly, show how each item of information can best be communicated to the expectant parents. An invaluable appendix is provided containing useful addresses (including those of international associations connected with the subject) and lists of necessary equipment such as slides and films, and where these may be obtained. A chapter entitled 'Some new ideas' has been added to this latest edition; it describes recent changes in labour ward procedure, and shows how these can affect the physiotherapist's preparation schemes.

Index

Abdominal muscles, 29, 31, 40
  exercise programme, 96
    in puerperium, 105
    in water, 123–124
  postnatal care, 32, 33
  Valsalva manoeuvre and, 65
Active Birth Movement, 14, 93
Acupuncture, 15, 130–139, 169, 182, 183, 184
  application technique, 131–132
  auricular points, 132–133
  historical aspects, 130–131
  in labour, 133–136
  opioid peptide release and, 136–137
Adductors, 112
Ambulant labour, 42, 43, 103–104, 181
Anorectal incontinence, idiopathic, 34
Antenatal classes, 103, 185
  abdominal muscle exercise, 96
  ACPOG physiotherapists and, 7, 8, 9
  back care, 76–77
  breathing awareness, 100
  historical aspects, 3
  learning to surrender, 64, 65
  postural exercises, 97–99, 100–103
  relaxation, 95, 99–100
  in swimming pool, see Aquatic antenatal classes
  TENS, 146–149
  in Western Australia, 22, 23, 28–31
Anthropoid pelvis, 41
Apgar score, 59, 62, 148
Aquatic antenatal classes, 108, 124–126
  body awareness, 117–119
  exercise goals, 117
  instructing team, 115–116
  organisational aspects, 115–117
  pool depth, 116–117
  posture and, 113
  relaxation, 119–20
  shaping up exercises, 120–124
  water temperature, 116
Association of Chartered Physiotherapists in Obstetrics and Gynaecology (ACPOG), 5–6, 172
  incontinence treatment, 16
  post-registration course, 5, 6–7
  promotional aspects, 13
  research by members, 12–13
  specialist physiotherapist's role, 7–8
  training for midwives, 9, 12
Association of Continence Advisors, 172
Association Nationale Natation et Maternité (ANNM), 107–108
  aims, 108–109

Back care, 94
  chair design and, 94
  preconceptual, 11, 16, 76, 89
  in pregnancy, 26, 28, 81, 82, 84
    programme for, 76–78
  prophylaxis in Western Australia, 26, 28
Back pain/backache, 16, 69–90, 105, 181
  assessment, 79–81
  exercise and, 81, 88
  fatigue-associated, 70
  heat treatment, 81, 87
  hormonal effects on connective tissue and, 70, 72–75
  incidence in pregnancy, 69
  interferential therapy, 82
  joint mobility and, 74, 75
  in labour, 44
  management, 78–79
  manipulation, 81, 82, 84–86, 183
  massage, 81, 87–88
  objective examination, 80–81

187

Back pain/backache (cont'd)
  pelvic support, 81, 83–84
  postnatal assessment/treatment, 33
  postural adaptation to pregnancy
    and, 71–72
  pregnancy-associated,
    signs/symptoms, 79, 80
  prophylaxis, see Back care
  psychological aspects, 75
  rest, 81, 82–83
  short-wave diathermy, 82, 87
  stirrups for delivery and, 58
  stress-related, 75–76, 83
  swimming and, 88, 113
  TENS, 81, 86–87
  traction, 81, 82, 86
  treatment modalities, 81–82
  weight gain and, 70–71
Bed-rest, 81, 82–83
Biofeedback, 169
Birth attendants, 45–46, 52–53, 64
  TENS and, 149
Birth chair, 59
Bladder, 153–154
  neurological control, 157
  training, 168–169
Blood pressure, 109, 115, 116
Blood sugar, 115, 117
Body awareness, 14, 93
  aquatic antenatal classes, 117–119
  back care and, 78, 84
  breathing, see Breathing awareness
  exercise programme, 100–103
  in first stage, 103–104
  pelvic floor muscles, 97
  postural sensitivity, 14, 94
  puerperium, 104–106
  relaxation, 14, 95
  in second stage, 104
Breath holding for delivery, 104, 124
Breathing awareness, 26, 28, 93,
    95–96
  exercise programme, 100
  in first stage, 104
Breathing, controlled patterns, 4, 5,
    14, 57, 59–61, 96
Breathing, spontaneous rhythm, 60
  antenatal swimming programme and,
    112
Bupivacaine, 129

Cardiovascular body changes, 109–110
  swimming and, 110
Carus, curve of, 41, 59
Cervical dilatation, pain and, 43–44

Chartered Society of Physiotherapy, 4
  ACPOG post-registration course, 5
  Education Subcommittee and, 12
  postgraduate acupuncture course, 15
  statement on working together in
    psychophysical preparation for
    childbirth, 10
Coccyx, 42
Cortisols, endogenous, 70

Delivery position, 14, 58, 104, 181,
    184
  aboriginal women, 43
  antenatal preparation, 93, 96
  gravity-assisted, 42, 43, 58, 97
  squatting, see Squatting
  supine, 58, 104
Diaphragm, 110, 112
Diastasis of rectus abdominis, 29, 32,
    96, 122
Diastasis of symphysis pubis, 29
Diuretics, 164, 165
Dyspareunia, 33, 35

Emepronium bromide, 168
Endorphins, 136, 137
  massage and, 88
  production in labour, 44, 55
Enkephalins, 136, 137
Epidural anaesthesia, 45, 129
  endogenous oxytocin release and, 61
  forceps rate and, 13, 15, 61
Episiotomy
  forced straining in second stage and,
    62–63
  pelvic floor function following, 13,
    162
Evolutionary aspects, 40, 41, 180
Exercise, 93
  abdominal muscles, 96, 105,
    123–124
  aims related to childbirth, 96
  antenatal, 30–31, 100–103, 183
  aquatic programme, 120–124
  back pain treatment, 81, 88
  pelvic floor muscles, 96–97
  postnatal, 33–34, 105
External urethral sphincter, 155

Faradism, 35, 169
Father, prospective, 46
Fembrace, 83, 85
Fetal head rotation, 52, 55
Flavoxate, 168

Forced pushing, 97, 104
  episiotomy, and, 62–63
Forceps delivery, 152
  epidural anaesthesia and, 13, 15, 61
  pelvic floor function following, 162

Gynaecoid pelvis, 41
Gynaecological care in Western
        Australia, 22, 34–35
  in service training, 36
  treatment modalities, 35

Health Visitors Association, 9, 10
Heat treatment for back pain, 81, 87
Hormonal changes of pregnancy, 93,
        94, 96, 97, 113
  effects on connective tissue, 70,
        72–75
Hyperlordosis, 113, 118, 120, 122
Hypertension, 114, 115
Hyperventilation, 5, 111, 112
Hypnosis, 15–16, 169
Hysterectomy, 168

Imipramine, 168
Incontinence clinic, 7
Incontinence urinary, 105, 151–173,
        179, 180
  bladder training, 168–169
  childbearing and, 152–153
  classification, 159
  definition, 151
  diuretic use and, 164, 165
  drug therapy, 168
  management, 166, 167
  overflow, 160–161
  pelvic floor re-education, 169–172
  prevalence, 151
  prevention, 11, 27, 164–166
  reflex, 160
  sites of lesions, 157
  stress, 34, 159–160
    aetiology, 161–163
    mechanism, 163–164
  surgery, 166, 168
  treatment, 8, 12, 16, 27, 168
  urge, 160, 168
  urodynamic studies, 159
Insomnia, 114
Inspiratory capacity, 110
Interferential therapy, 12, 35, 169
International Back Pain Society, 89
International Continence Society, 172,
        179

Lying, 94, 97–98

3M Tenzcare, 144, 145
Manipulation, 81, 82, 84–86
Massage, 104, 114, 120
  of baby, 34
  back pain and, 81, 87–88
  dyspareunia and, 35
Mastitis, 33
McGill Pain Questionnaire, 39, 47,
        48–49
Microceptor II, 144, 145
Micturition, neurological control, 157
Moulding of fetal head, 40, 41

Naloxone, 137
Neuromuscular control, see Relaxation
Neuropeptides, 136
Non-forced pushing, 62, 97, 104

Obstetric Association of Chartered
        Physiotherapists, 5
Oestrogen, 70
Opioid peptides, 137
Oxytocin
  epidural anaesthesia and, 61
  maternal position and, 59
  proprioceptor stimulation and, 61

Pain intensity, 39
Pain, labour, 39–55, 63, 64, 183
  anatomical aspects, 39–42
  antenatal training and, 46–55
  anterior, 141
  assessment, 133, 134
  back, 44
  fetal position and, 50, 51
  historical aspects, 39
  ischaemic uterus, 45
  measurement, 39, 47, 48–49
  observational study, 46–55
    pain questionnaire, 47, 48–49
    pain rating index, 49
    research method, 47–49
    results, 50–54
  overworking uterus, 45
  physiological factors, 43
  posterior, 141
  psychological aspects, 45–46
  stretch/pressure, 44
  support persons and, 46, 52–53
  suprapubic, 142, 148
Pain relief, 14–15, 54
  acupuncture see Acupuncture
  drugs, 129–130

Pain relief (*cont'd*)
  epidural anaestheisa, 13, 15, 45, 61, 129
  TENS, *see* Transcutaneous electrical nerve stimulation (TENS)
Pain scales, 47, 48–49, 53
Pain threshold, 39
Pain tolerance, 14, 39
Pelvic floor, 28, 40, 179
  anatomical aspects, 155–156
  antenatal preparation in swimming pool, 112, 113, 117, 124
  assessment of muscle function, 170–171
  body awareness and, 97
  delivery position and, 13, 97
  exercise, 96–97, 103, 112, 113
  for senior citizens, 38
  fetal head rotation and, 42
  forceps delivery, damage and, 13, 152
  functional aspects, 156–157
  incontinence prophylaxis, 11
  non-forced pushing and, 97
  post-natal aspects, 32, 33, 96–97, 105
  research by specialist physiotherapists, 12–13
  stretch receptor stimulation in second stage, 61
  Valsalva manoeuvre and, 65
Pelvic floor re-education, 16, 34, 169–172
  assessment of muscle strength, 170–171
  electrical treatment, 169
  exercise, 170–172
Pelvic inflammatory disease, 8
Pelvic rocking, 100, 104, 112
Pelvic support, 81, 83–84
Pelvis, 72–78, 184
  anatomical types, 41
  evolutionary aspects, 40
  joint mobility, 42–43
Perionometer, 11, 171–172
Pethidine, 15, 129, 130
Postnatal exercise, 96, 184
  ACPOG physiotherapists and, 9
  historical aspects, 9
  in swimming pool, 126–128
  in Western Australia, 22, 23, 31–34
Posture, 94, 113
  abdominal muscles and, 96
  antenatal swimming and, 113
  back pain and, 78, 81, 84

changes in pregnancy, 29, 70–72, 113
  evolutionary aspects, 40
  exercises, 97–99, 104–106
  lying, 94, 97–98
  in puerperium, 105
  relaxation, 105
  sitting, 94, 99
  standing, 94, 98
  stress-related changes, 76
Post-registration courses, 3, 11–12, 17
  ACPOG, 5, 6–7
Preconceptual clinics, 11, 93
Progesterone, 70
Propantheline, 168
Psychological changes, 114
Psychoprophylaxis, 4–5, 96
Psychotherapy, 169
Pubic symphysis
  changes in pregnancy, 73
  diastasis, 29
  mobility, 42, 72
  relaxin and, 74, 75
Pulsed short wave treatment, 8
Pushing in second stage
  endogenous oxytocin release and, 61
  establishment of expulsive urge and, 61, 64
  forced, 57, 61, 62, 104
    episiotomy and, 62–63
  spontaneous efforts, 62, 97, 104
  Valsalva manoeuvre and, 62, 63

Q.B. TENS, 144, 145

Relaxation, 14, 26, 65, 93, 95, 183
  body awareness and, 78, 84
  exercise programme, 99–100
  in first stage, 104
  historical aspects, 3, 4
  Mitchell Method, 28, 31, 78, 84, 95, 99
  postnatal, 33, 105
  TENS and, 147
  in water, 112, 117, 119–200
Relaxin, 70, 74–75, 182
Residual volume, 110
Respiratory alkalosis, 111, 112
Respiratory changes in pregnancy, 110
Royal College of Midwives, 9, 10

Sacro-iliac joint, 29, 42, 72, 98, 181
  mobility, 72–73, 74
  strain
    due to stirrups delivery, 58
    due to weight gain, 71, 77

Second stage, 182
 breathing, 104, 111–112, 113, 124
 delivery in water, 112
 fetal parameters, maternal effort
   and, 62–63
 metabolic acidosis, 111
 position, *see* Delivery position
 pushing, *see* Pushing in second stage
 preparation in swimming pool,
   112–113
 respiratory alkalosis, 111, 112
 Valsalva manoeuvre, 62, 63, 65
Self-control in labour, 57, 63, 64, 65
Short-wave diathermy, 35
Sitting, 94, 99
Squatting, 104
 antenatal practice, 93, 102
 in birth chair, 59
 control of pelvic floor and, 163, 165
Standing, 94, 98
Standing up, 98
Stress, 95
 controlled breathing and, 96
 postural effects, 76
Stretching exercises, 4, 12
Supine hypotension, 58
Supine position, 58, 61, 104
Swimming, 16, 88, 107
 cardiovascular effects, 110
 contra-indications in pregnancy, 114
 respiration and, 112–113
 see also Aquatic antenatal classes

Team approach, 9–10
 aquatic antenatal classes, 115–116
Tidal volume, 110
Traction, 81, 86
Transcutaneous electrical nerve
   stimulation (TENS), 15,
   141–149, 180, 182
 antenatal instruction, 146–149
 batteries, 145
 biphasic wave forms, 144
 birth attendant and, 149
 contra-indications, 149

dual channel systems, 143
electrodes, 145
fetal monitoring and, 148
historical aspects, 143
history of use in labour, 141–143
informed consent form, 147
in labour, 143–146
models, 144

Ultrasound, 35
Upright position
 delivery, *see* Delivery position
 first stage, 103–104
 pelvic floor muscles and, 13
Urethra, 154–155
Urodynamic investigations, 7, 159
Uterus, labour pain and, 45

Vagina, evolutionary aspects, 40–41
Valsalva manoeuvre, 62, 63, 65
Varicose veins, 110, 122
Visual Analogue Scale, 39, 47, 49, 53,
   130, 133, 143, 147
Vital capacity, 110, 112

Well Women's Clinics, 172
 back pain prevention, 11, 76
Western Australia, service in, 19–38
 aims of service, 20–21
 antenatal programme, 22, 23, 28–31
 clinical programmes, 22–23
 gynaecological service, 22, 34–35
 in-service training, 35–36
 inter-professional liaison, 27–28
 isolated women's needs, 25–26
 language/cultural barriers, 27
 monitoring service, 24–25
 postgraduate diploma, 36–37
 postnatal classes, 22, 23, 31–34
 postregistration courses, 17
 procedure manual, 20, 21
 rural industries, special needs of,
   26–27
 special interest group, 37